THE HEALTH CARE SUPERVISOR'S HANDBOOK

Norman Metzger

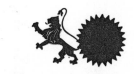

Aspen Systems Corporation
Germantown, Maryland
1978

Library of Congress Cataloging in Publication Data

Metzger, Norman, 1924—

The health care supervisor's handbook.

Includes bibliographical references and index.
1. Health facilities— Personnel management.
2. Supervision of employees. I. Title.
RA971.35.M46   658.3'7'3621   78-12513
ISBN 0-89443-078-5

Library of Congress Catalog Card Number: 78-12513
ISBN: 0-89443-078-5
Printed in the United States of America

5

Table of Contents

Foreword

Supervisors will readily agree with me when I state that the responsibility of supervising other people is complex, undervalued, and misunderstood. I have tried to clear up some of the misunderstandings and present "keys" to successful supervision. At all times I have recognized the supervisor's critical contribution to the delivery of health services.

I have conducted a thorough review of the literature and am indebted to all the researchers and authors from whom I have drawn. Once again, I wish to acknowledge the invaluable contribution of Dr. Leslie M. Slote to my thinking and writing in the area of management science. Ours has been a relationship and friendship over two-and-a-half decades.

I have reconsidered my own experiences over some thirty years of managing, teaching, and writing. This was a particularly rewarding endeavor. My first five books (three coauthored with Dr. Dennis Pointer) dealt with labor relations and personnel administration. It is clear to me that the real job of labor and employee relations is done on a day-to-day basis by the first-line supervisor and the department head. I address this study—this "how-to" manual—to all of you who get the job done.

I wish to acknowledge, as I have in my other books, the contribution of Marlin (Bud) Cruse to the final work presented here. He was the "supervisor" of this effort.

I dedicate this book to the many competent members of the management team—especially those first-line supervisors—at The Mount Sinai Medical Center.

Norman Metzger

"The great characteristic of our time is that we know everything important about human nature that there is to know. Yet never has there been an age in which so little knowledge is securely possessed, so little a part of the common understanding. The reason is precisely the advance of specialization, the impossibility of making safe general statements, which has led to a general imbecility. What I would like to do in these few pages is to run the risk of simple-mindedness in order to make some dent in the unintended imbecility brought about by specialization and its mountains of fact. Even if I succeed poorly, it seems like a worthwhile barter. In such a stifling and crushing scientific epoch someone has to be willing to play the fool in order to relieve the general myopia."

Ernest Becker, THE DENIAL OF DEATH

Chapter 1

The Supervisor as Manager

ORGANIZATIONAL ANALYSIS

Throughout the years I have been lecturing to first-line supervisors and middle managers in the classrooms of major universities, in the board rooms of hospitals, and at meetings of various associations. A single question comes up again and again: What is a supervisor? The question is easy to answer; it is far more important to discover the reason the question is asked.

To define a supervisor we can refer to two sources: The National Labor Relations Act (NLRA) and the Fair Labor Standards Act (FLSA). Supervisors are specifically excluded from the provisions of the NLRA through Section 14(a). Section 2(11) states that:

> The term "supervisor" means any individual having authority in the interests of the employer to hire, transfer, suspend, lay off, recall, promote, discharge, assign, reward or discipline other employees, or responsibility to direct them or to adjust their grievances or effectively to recommend such action if in connection with the foregoing, the exercise of such authority is not of a merely routine or clerical nature, but requires the use of independent judgment.

The Fair Labor Standards Act specifically excludes supervisors from its coverage and, therefore, from the requirement of providing premium compensation for overtime. A supervisor is defined as follows:

Under the Fair Labor Standards Act the term "employee employed in a bona fide executive capacity" means any employee:

a. Whose primary duty consists of the management of the enterprise in which he is employed or of a customarily recognized department or subdivision thereof; and

b. Who customarily and regularly directs the work of two or more other employees therein; and

c. Who has the authority to hire or fire other employees or whose suggestions and recommendations as to the hiring or firing and as to the advancement and promotion or any other change of status of other employees will be given particular weight; and

d. Who customarily and regularly exercises discretionary powers; and

e. Who does not devote more than 20% or in the case of an employee of a retail or service establishment, who does not devote as much as 40% of his hours of work in the work week to activities which are not directly and closely related to the performance of the work described in paragraphs (a) through (d) above.

The term "employee employed in a bona fide administrative capacity" means any employee:

a. Whose primary duty consists of either:

1. The performance of office or nonmanual work directly related to management policies or general business operations of his employer or his employer's customers or

2. The performance of functions in the administration of a school system or educational establishment or institution or of a department or subdivision thereof in work directly related to the academic instruction or training carried on therein; and

b. Who customarily and regularly exercises discretion and independent judgment, and

c. 1. Who regularly and directly assists a proprietor or an employee employed in a bona fide executive or administrative capacity, or

2. Who performs under only general supervision work along specialized or technical lines requiring special training, experience or knowledge or

3. Who executes under only general supervision special assignments and tasks; and

d. Who does not devote more than 20% or, in the case of an employee of a retail or service establishment who does not devote as much as 40% , of his hours worked in the work week to activities which are not directly and closely related to the performance of the work described in paragraphs (a) through (c) above.

More important than this mechanical definition is the true state of affairs in which many people with the title of supervisor do not "feel" like supervisors. They do not feel like supervisors because they are not clear about their place in the hierarchy or are not given appropriate recognition.

Several observations about supervisors can serve as the cornerstone of this book:

1. The supervisor is the person in the middle. The supervisor represents the administration to the employees and represents the employees to the administration.

2. In a union certification election more employees vote for or against their immediate supervisor than for or against the institution itself as personified by the top administration.

3. In almost every instance the basic difference between a supervisor and a worker is the supervisor's responsibility to get work done through other people.

4. In order to get work done through other people, supervisors must improve their skills in

a. interviewing,

b. evaluating performance,

c. communicating for change, and

d. disciplining positively.

This "how-to" book will present usable, understandable, and universal suggestions on building effective work teams with or without top administration's support. Too often supervisors listen to obviously sensible and workable techniques of dealing with their employees and respond "that may be okay at your hospital, but it just won't go at ours." What they are saying is the lifestyle of their organization presents negative forces that mitigate against positive supervisory techniques.

THE NEW BREED OF SUPERVISOR

All persons in formal control over others are supervisors regardless of their high or low status in the hierarchy. Line supervisors are generally supposed to have a "bossing" relationship to the workers, while functional supervisors are subject matter specialists who exercise a larger undefined influence sometimes referred to as "the authority of ideas."[1]

It is a paradox that as time has passed, the job of the first-line supervisor has not been simplified, but rather has become more complex. As a supervisor, you must be a respected leader of the rank and file employees; you often need technical know-how of the specific area you supervise; you must be able to plan the work; and you must, of course, deal with interpersonal relationships. You are the person in the middle. It is clear that no less than five different roles come into play almost every day you report to work. You supervise and train the employees in your department; you are responsible for implementing ideas that you have generated or that originate from the staff specialists; you have peer relationships with other supervisors; and you report to someone—you relate to your boss as your employees relate to you. Not the least of the roles you play is that of mediator, whether it be in a union shop where you interface with the shop steward or in a nonunion shop where you deal directly with your employees.[2]

In the past, supervisors have been chosen on the basis of either strength or technical know-how. In that era the biggest bully could well have moved into the position designated as supervisor. Very often a supervisor was selected on the basis of technical know-how. He or she was the best at whatever was being done mechanically, physically, or cerebrally.

In the last several decades, research has indicated there is not a one-to-one relationship between technical proficiency and supervisory skills. The "art" of supervision has been reshaped into the "science" of supervision. Once we dispensed with the myth that the best worker could become the best supervisor, we had to address ourselves to the myth that "good supervisors are born, not made." There is little doubt today that almost every technique of supervision can be learned. These basic principles more often than not can be transferred from workplace to workplace. Indeed, the backbone of supervisory techniques is pure and simple common sense.

The new breed of supervisors must master the art and science of consultation. Two-way communication, with a feedback loop, is the hallmark of today's successful supervisor. If you are to do your job properly, gain the respect and admiration of your subordinates, and obtain recognition and rewards from your superiors, then you must see beyond the day-to-day details of the job and develop your ability to understand the motivations of your subordinates; learn how to speak their language, master techniques of introducing change in the face of resistance, control subjective evaluation and determination, and replace subjectivity with dependence on facts and logic.

Rather than get caught up in academic phrases and labels, most of the researchers involved in supervisor-subordinate relationships seem to address their studies to two diametrically opposed styles of supervision—supervisors who are employee centered and supervisors who are production centered.

The Institute for Social Research at the University of Michigan has conducted numerous studies in an attempt to find out what makes an organization tick and, more specifically, how the principles and practices of leadership bear directly on the productivity and job satisfaction of various groups. These studies concluded that:

1. It is not necessarily true that a favorable attitude among employees toward the company will result in increased productivity.

2. When comparing people under general supervision (where the goal to be accomplished is clear and the employees are given leeway in accomplishing it) with persons under close supervision (where the supervisor is constantly in attendance and permits little leeway for the subordinates), those groups under *close supervision* tend to be associated with *low productivity* while those under more *general supervision* show *higher productivity*.

3. Supervisors of high-productivity groups more often report that they are kept informed of developments than do supervisors of low-productivity groups.

4. When work groups with the highest and lowest morale were asked to describe what their supervisors did, workers in low-morale groups mentioned just as often as workers in high-morale groups that their supervisors performed such production-centered tasks as "enforces the rules," "arranges work and makes work assignments," and "supplies men with materials and tools." But the high-morale groups mentioned much more frequently than the low-morale groups such employee-centered functions as "recommends promotions and pay increases," "informs men on what is happening in the company," "keeps men posted on how well they are doing," and "hears complaints and grievances."

5. There is a marked relationship between worker morale and how strongly employees feel that their boss is interested in discussing work problems with the work group.

6. The high-production groups show greater group loyalty and greater group pride than do the low-production groups.
7. When supervisors were asked, "How does your section compare with other sections in the way the men help each other on the job?", the answer showed a marked relationship to group productivity. Supervisors of high-production groups reported much more often than supervisors of low-production groups that their workers helped one another in getting the work done.[3]

Likert concludes that when a supervisor treats subordinates as human beings, the result is greater group loyalty and pride. He states that when supervisors stay sufficiently close to their workers to be able to see work-related problems through employees' eyes, the supervisors are better able to develop good group loyalty. Supervisors who can empathize with workers can translate employee needs to top administration and thereby help arrive at policy decisions that are realistic and satisfactory to both the administration and the employees.

An effective supervisor must understand employee motivations and needs. Study after study has shown that supervisors and the people they supervise do not see eye to eye on what workers want most. The average supervisor replies that good wages, job security, and promotion are the worker's basic desires. On the other hand, workers consistently reply that their basic desires are "full appreciation of work done," "feeling in on things," and "sympathetic help on personal problems." Simply stated, there are two pay systems operative in every institution. The normal pay system is based on competitive wages and fair differentials within the institution, resulting in an adequate and satisfactory paycheck; *the other pay system deals with employee motivation.*

A most interesting study by Frederick Herzberg revealed the duality of a person's nature. The study was designed to search out people's needs, to test the concept that a person has two sets of needs—a need as an animal to avoid pain and a need as a human being to grow psychologically. The participants in the study were professionals. They were asked to recall a time when they had felt exceptionally good about their jobs and the reasons for these feelings. They were also asked if these feelings of satisfaction in regard to their work had affected their performance, their personal relationships, and their well-being. The study concluded that engineers and accountants rated as the strongest *determiners of job satisfaction:* achievements, recognition, work itself, responsibility, and advancement. The last three factors were more important to a lasting change of attitudes than the first two factors. The major *dissatisfiers* were company policy and administration, supervision, salary, interpersonal relations, and working conditions. The *satisfiers* relate to what the person does, while the *dissatisfiers* relate to the situation in which he does it. The satisfier factors were named the *motivators;* the dissatisfier factors were named the *hygiene.* Herzberg concluded that the motivators were effective in promoting superior performance and effort.[4]

To fully understand why appreciation, recognition, and consultation are far more important to employees than wages, let us look quickly at Maslow's hierarchical structure of importance. Maslow points out that there are basically five levels of needs. The lowest are the physiological ① needs: the need for air, food, and health. When these needs are reasonably satisfied, they no longer act as motivators to behavior. At the second ② level is the need for safety, for protection against danger and threat, for the fairest possible break. If the employee is confident that his safety needs are met, these too are no longer motivators, but if he feels threatened or dependent, he is motivated to seek security. At the next ③ level are the social needs. These needs are best typified by the drive to belong, to be part of a purposeful group. We then move to the ego needs. ④ These are the need for self-esteem, for self-confidence, for status. These are rarely satisfied and have a far greater effect on motivation. At the ⑤ fifth level is the need for self-fulfillment, the need for realizing one's own potential.[5]

You, as a supervisor, must accept the fact that by improved managerial practices and attention to the proper utilization of people and technology, you can increase the satisfaction and productivity of the people who work for you. This is made clear by much of the theory and research on organizational motivation, satisfaction, and productivity. Such research indicates that people bring to the work area different mental and physical abilities. Supervisors must deal with varying personalities and varying levels of experience.

Need fulfillment or frustration produces either constructive or defensive behavior. How often have you noted tensions in employees who seem to be dissatisfied by their work? Such dissatisfaction produces behavior designed to relieve that tension. Employees whose needs are not met become defensive; they employ defense mechanisms such as withdrawal, aggression, substitution, or compensation. You must have seen employees who do very little talking; they seem withdrawn and you have great difficulty in communicating with them. Other dissatisfied employees channel their frustration into constructive behavior by looking outside the work area for fulfillment. They join clubs, teams, or unions. Defensive behavior may work against the goals of the department and of the institution. Dissatisfaction on the job exacts a high cost. It produces friction on the job, low productivity, high absenteeism, excessive turnover, and, of course, strikes. Many employees seek more satisfaction from their work than is available to them under present managerial structures. There is little question that employee motivation results in increased productivity and higher efficiency. Such motivation can be enhanced by a supervisory style that encompasses the knowledge and appreciation of employee motives.

A relationship between a supervisor and workers which includes mutual understanding and agreement on goals and rewards is an ideally effective one. Supervisors must be willing to move from authority-obedience styles of supervision to involvement-participation-commitment styles. Supervisors are responsible for getting results from their work team. Therefore, they must demand such results. However, demanding results does not necessarily guarantee results. More and more evidence has been produced to indicate that the old authority-obedience approach is not result oriented. Yet the involvement-participation-commitment style of supervision is difficult and complex. The new approach involves reaching consensus on what is the real problem to be solved in any given case, listening for reservations and doubts rather than for signs of compliance, getting people to express their different views, and dealing with conflicts in an open and candid way.[6]

To repeat an earlier statement, research and experience clearly indicate that a supervisor is indeed able to meet the needs of employees and thereby make them more productive. Although there is no one sure way to make employees more efficient, there is a central theme that weaves through the mass of research and literature on this subject. This central theme which found its way through the works of McGregor, Mayo, and Herzberg and was emblazoned in the singular study, *Work in America,* points an accusing finger at the typical organization. Employees who start a new job bring with them a caring attitude and a high level of motivation. The subsequent lack of productivity and efficiency is usually caused by the organization, which by its inherent noncaring style destroys an employee's natural desire to care about work and to do it well.

It falls then to the supervisor to restructure the work situation for the employee. This restructuring includes an objective review of work content with an eye toward enrichment, redesign, and broadening of responsibilities. This is necessary because worker motivation derives from the task itself. In addition to the challenge of improving the job, attention must be directed toward improving the environment. Recognition is necessary at every level of the organization. Communication is just as important to the porter as it is to the surgeon. Everyone wants to be in on things. Employees want to know what the supervisor is thinking and what management is thinking and planning. They want to feel that management knows that they are there—that they are not invisible. Alienation and frustration will develop if employees feel nobody is listening or paying attention to their needs. The wise supervisor who directs his or her attention toward maximizing opportunities for effective work teams will keep these conclusions in mind and not be confused by long ingrained beliefs and myths which are counterproductive in an attempt to get the job done.

Boyd and Scanlan offer four key factors that aid new supervisors moving into the world of management:

1. *Job knowledge.* Being technically equipped for the type of work you will supervise will be of immeasurable assistance in bolstering your confidence; your subordinates will recognize that you know what you are talking about.

2. *Assistance from others.* Don't be shy. Ask your superior or your peers for any support and advice that you need. It is not a sign of weakness.

3. *Good education.* Much of what you do involves communications, paperwork, and arithmetic. If you have educated yourself, you are a step ahead in the supervisory world. But remember, what counts is the quality, not the quantity, of your schooling.

4. *Desire to succeed.* There is no substitute for the will to do a good job. You have been selected for the responsibility and there is no reason why you shouldn't succeed if you try hard enough.[7]

The National Management Association made a study of 68 companies to determine why some supervisors fail:

1. poor general relations with workers or with other management people,

2. individual shortcomings such as lack of initiative and emotional instability,

3. lack of understanding of the management point of view,

4. unwillingness to spend the necessary time and effort to improve,

5. lack of skill in planning and organizing work, and

6. inability to adjust to new and changing conditions.[8]

The mark of the good supervisor is the ability to develop sound interpersonal relationships with workers and with other management people. In order to do this, the supervisor must respond to different types of organizational situations on the basis of the differences in employee personalities. The successful supervisor is the *people-centered supervisor.*

This type of supervisor understands the needs of various employees under his or her jurisdiction.

The supervisor is often the only individual in the institution dealing daily with today's problems. He or she is often many people rolled up in one: counselor to employees, interpreter of the institution's policies, and implementer of the institution's programs. The supervisor must deal with staff people, medical people, top-level administrative people, union representatives, and often the public. This obviously requires a person with a grasp for differences. Supervisors must be able to adapt to new situations and a wide range of personalities.

First-line supervisors are the people on the firing line. Their prime responsibility is to develop their subordinates into an efficient production-oriented team, while at the same time keep friction at a minimum, satisfaction at a maximum, and achieve optimum stability. I cannot think of a more difficult position in the organization than that of the first-line supervisor.

The supervisory role encompasses a broad range of responsibilities:

1. Supervisors are the immediate leaders of designated segments of the work force.
2. Supervisors are day-to-day decision makers.
3. Supervisors must plan.
4. Supervisors must organize the work, the work area, and the workers.
5. Supervisors are responsible for setting up conditions that provide for maximum motivation of the work force.
6. Supervisors must counsel employees on job-related and other problems.
7. Supervisors must be communicators.
8. Supervisors are trainers.
9. Finally, most difficult and possibly the most important, supervisors must be "change agents."

SOME TOUGH QUESTIONS FOR SUPERVISORY ASPIRANTS

I have often felt that it takes a great deal more than the obvious ingredients of desire, integrity, and technical know-how to be a supervisor. Recently I came across a list of questions set forth by Black and Black to ascertain if you really have what it takes to be a supervisor. They are worth repeating here.

1. Are you able to take the loss of credit? You will be faced with the

problem of your idea showing up as someone else's brilliant stroke of imagination.

2. Are you susceptible to the frustrations of communications break-downs? Do you lose your temper when "you didn't get the word?"

3. Are you big enough to absorb the blame for a subordinate's mistake? You are going to have to be if you intend to put together a successful and efficient team.

4. Are you unable to cope with disappointment? There are going to be many disappointments ahead, but the "successful/unsuccessful super-visor" has to control resentment and move on to future successes.

5. Can you work for an unreasonable boss? This question is a real soul-searcher. Too often supervisors—those that do not make it—undercut their superior. You often must look beyond your own agenda and at-tempt to understand actions of your superior that appear to be unreasonable.

6. Can you separate your life off the job from your life on the job? This may be the most difficult requirement for a manager, but it is the mark of the successful and experienced supervisor.

7. Can you keep pushing when there is no penalty for taking it easy? This is the test of true leadership; motivation to succeed comes from within.[9]

There is no question that supervisors face frustrating circumstances on a daily basis. Too often those at the top have lost touch with the problems and frustrations of the first-line supervisor. More often than not you find yourself in an organization reluctant to share decision making, an organization that does not understand or appreciate your contribution, an organization that does not seem to be able to differentiate between productive employees and nonproductive employees. It takes a great deal to succeed in the face of these obstacles, but successful managers seem to have the personality for the job.

THE SUCCESSFUL SUPERVISOR

There has been a great deal of research regarding the desirable traits indicative of the successful manager. You find such words as decisive, in-formed, creative—but more important is a general behavioral pattern that has emerged from opinions, observations, tests and intensive research into the actual process of supervision. The following list of job behaviors seems consistent with that research:

1. Successful managers manage work instead of people.
2. They plan and organize effectively.
3. They set goals realistically.
4. They derive decisions by group consensus, but accept responsibility for them.
5. They delegate frequently and effectively.
6. They rely on others for help in solving problems.
7. They communicate effectively.
8. They are a stimulus to action.
9. They coordinate effectively.
10. They cooperate with others.
11. They show consistent and dependable behavior.
12. They win gracefully.
13. They express hostility tactfully.[10]

Of course it is rarely possible to be all things to all people. The job of the supervisor is indeed broad in its demands and complex in its challenges. My own observations lead me to conclude that more often than not, the supervisor who has an efficient department is sensitive to three basic areas that affect the quality of employee performance. These areas are participation, communication, and motivation. Participation is accomplished by encouraging subordinates to offer suggestions about work flow and working conditions. It is enhanced by delegating responsibility. You maximize participation by setting up an atmosphere where subordinates can offer ideas, react to your ideas without fear of retribution, and participate in group decisions.

The hallmark of effective communication is the feedback loop. There must be two-way communication; there must be a system that permits and encourages "checking" messages for understanding. Communication is enhanced by a permissive atmosphere where *cooperation rather than competition is encouraged*. Effective communication is built upon consultation and collaboration.

Motivation is at the heart of the modern manager's job. The successful supervisor needs to become conscious of three factors: (a) the needs and policies of the institution, (b) the needs and interests of the workers, and (c) the supervisor's own purposes and goals.

Here is a simple list of recommended supervisory practices:

1. Keep employees informed of work requirements.
2. Let employees know where they stand.
3. Obtain maximum participation and strive for maximum communication where changes are indicated.

4. Help employees improve and broaden their skills.

5. Compliment employees for a job well done.

6. Provide the opportunity for group and individual participation for solving operational problems.

7. Treat all members of the group as equals.

8. Delegate responsibilities and encourage the acceptance of such responsibilities by all members of the work team.

9. Understand each employee's job and clarify the importance of each job in relation to the group.

10. Appreciate and attempt to solve and alleviate employees' problems, no matter how minute.

11. Help the individual understand the basic reasons for management's thinking on things that they are required to do.

CHECKLIST FOR SUPERVISORS

To help you build more effective work teams, we will deal in subsequent chapters with interviewing skills, evaluating skills, communication skills, disciplining skills, and a review of measurement techniques. But before we go any further, I have prepared a list of questions that require you to take a look at yourself as a supervisor and give you an advance look at what is ahead in the remaining pages of this book.[11]

1. Do you have a thorough understanding of the institution's goals and your part in meeting the objectives of the institution and budget goals for your department? Do you have full confidence in their attainment?

2. Do you avoid confusion with a clear understanding of what is expected and how to do it?

3. Do you offer suggestions or constructive criticism to your immediate supervisor and ask for additional information when necessary?

4. Do you build team spirit and group pride by getting everyone into the act of setting goals and pulling together?

5. Are you always submerged in operational emergencies, or do you schedule time for meetings with your subordinates and with your superiors?

6. Do you encourage each of your employees to come up with suggestions about ways to improve things?

7. Do you make it easy for your people to approach you with job or personal problems?

8. Do you keep your employees informed on how they are doing?

9. Are you too busy with operational problems to be concerned with your employees' personal difficulties?

10. Do you give your employees a feeling of accomplishment by telling them how well they are doing in comparison with yesterday or last week or a month or a year ago?

11. Do you build individual employee confidence and praise good performance, or are you afraid of being accused of sentimentality, coddling, and soft-soaping?

12. Do you use personnel records and close observation to learn exactly which skills each employee has so that his or her best abilities may be used?

13. Do you let your people know how jobs are analyzed and evaluated and what the job rates and progressions are? Do you attempt to rotate people on different jobs to build up skills for individual flexibility within the group?

14. Do you train your people for better jobs?

15. Are you developing an understudy for your job?

16. Do you hold a good person down in one position because he or she may be indispensable there?

17. Do you take a chance on your people by letting them learn through mistakes, by showing a calm reaction and constructive approach to occasional failure, by encouraging them to stick their neck out without fear of the ax, and by instilling an atmosphere of confidence?

18. Do you use every opportunity to build up in your employees a sense of importance in their work?

19. Do you delegate responsibility to subordinates, or do you insist on keeping your hand in details?

20. Are you placing real responsibility on your subordinates and then holding them accountable?

21. Do you interfere with the jobs of subordinates or do you allow them to exercise discretion and judgment in making decisions?

22. Are you doing things to discourage your subordinates?

23. Are you aware of sources of discontentment or discouragement or frustration affecting your employees?

24. Do you listen to the ideas and reactions of subordinates with courtesy? If an idea is adopted or not accepted, do you explain why?

25. Do you usually praise in public, but criticize or reprove in private? Is criticism constructive?

26. Are you aware that a feeling of belonging builds self-confidence and makes people want to work harder than ever?

27. Do you ever say or do anything that detracts from the sense of personal dignity that each of your people has?

These are very difficult questions, but they must be reviewed. Your honest answers will give you a good picture of your present supervisory style.

Key Points for the Supervisor as a Manager

In this first chapter, it should have become obvious to you that the following key points will make you more effective as a supervisor:

1. You have more status than you think you have. Such status derives from employees' perception of their immediate supervisors. You are the "boss" to the average employee in your department.
2. You are often the person in the middle, but still you can arrive at a productive and efficient relationship with the people you supervise.
3. Consultation can be of enormous assistance to you in getting people to do their jobs.
4. Two-way communication is essential for the modern manager.
5. Successful supervision is not constant supervision. Know your people and give to each what is needed in the way of instruction, information, and evaluation.
6. Remember there are two pay systems: the normal pay system built on competitive wages and fair differentials, and the other pay system which includes appreciation, communication, and opportunity for fulfillment.
7. Many of your employees desire more challenging work. Productive and efficient employees should not be "hoarded" by the supervisor. Provide opportunities for advancement and more challenging work even if this means a transfer out of your department.
8. The supervisor who moves into higher positions in the institution is more often than not a people-centered supervisor. He or she has obtained results through appreciating and understanding employees' needs.
9. Participation is essential to the success of a work team. The supervisor achieves participation by encouraging subordinates to make suggestions. Such encouragement is enhanced by a nonjudgmental attitude toward suggestions and a willingness to explore the feasibility of all suggestions.
10. If you are going to succeed in the modern work arena—with its complex challenges produced by changes in our society, higher expectations from employees, and a more educated work group,

then you must move from a supervisory style anchored in authority-obedience to one based on involvement-participation-commitment.

NOTES

1. John M. Pfiffner, *The Supervision of Personnel: Human Relations and the Management of Men* (Englewood Cliffs, N.J.: Prentice-Hall, Inc., 2nd ed., 1958), pp. 6-7.

2. Lester R. Bittel, *What Every Supervisor Should Know* (New York: McGraw Hill Book Company, 2nd ed., 1968), p. 4.

3. Rensis Likert, *Motivation: The Core of Management, Personnel Series No. 155* (New York: American Management Association, 1953), pp. 3-20.

4. Frederick Herzberg, *Work and the Nature of Man* (Cleveland and New York: The World Publishing Company, 1966), pp. 71-76.

5. A. H. Maslow, *Motivation and Personality* (New York: Harper & Brothers, 2nd ed., 1970), Chapters 3-7.

6. Robert R. Blake and Jane Srygley Mouton, *The Grid for Supervisory Effectiveness* (Austin, Texas: Scientific Methods, Inc., 1975), p. 3.

7. Radford B. Boyd and Burt K. Scanlan, *Management Institute of the University of Wisconsin Survey of 215 First Line Supervisors* (Madison: University of Wisconsin, 1972).

8. Bittel, *op. cit.,* pp. 12-13.

9. James Menzies Black and Virginia Todd Black, *The Front Line Manager's Problem Solver* (New York: McGraw Hill Book Company, 1970), p. 8.

10. J. P. Campbell et al., *Managerial Behavior, Performance and Effectiveness* (New York: McGraw Hill Book Company, 1970), p. 8.

11. The author wishes to take special note of the contribution of Dr. Leslie M. Slote, Hartsdale, N.Y., who helped develop checklists similar to those presented here.

Chapter 2

How To Interview: First Step to Better Placement

Each new employee hired provides the supervisor with an opportunity to strengthen the effectiveness of the work team. Too often one hears supervisors complain that "the personnel department does the hiring." The final responsibility for hiring must lie with an employee's immediate supervisor. Given the importance of the employment interview, it is disturbing to note that most supervisors are not equipped to handle interviewing because of little understanding of and minimal training in interviewing techniques.

THE EFFECTIVE EMPLOYMENT INTERVIEW

It will help to review some key steps to follow in the employment interview. The supervisor who wishes to be effective in the employment interview should do the following:

1. Set a plan. Structure the interview to obtain maximum information and cover all necessary areas.

2. Review the job specification and/or job description. There is nothing more fatal to positive results than to enter the employment interview with scarce knowledge of the job requirements. If the personnel department has not provided you with a written description of the job, then write one yourself.

3. Don't begin the interview until you have reviewed the job application. Have the applicant wait outside your office while you review the application form, any tests administered by your personnel department, and any reference checks made in advance.

4. Pick the right place for an interview— it should be held in private. Limit phone calls that can disturb the applicant and interrupt your train of thought. Ensure that you have enough time (30 to 45 minutes).

5. Familiarize yourself with the five logical segments of the employment interview (warm-up stage, applicant talking stage, question stage, employer information stage, wind-up stage).

6. Keep in mind that it is not necessary for you to impress the applicant with the importance of your position. This means you are going to have to control the amount of time you talk as compared with the amount of time that the applicant is permitted to talk.

7. Watch the level of your language. Speak *to* the applicant in terms easy to understand, not above or beneath his or her level.

8. Watch your biases; don't let them get in the way of your ability to select the best qualified applicant.

9. Don't be hesitant about making notes; make a record of essential facts and judgments during and after the interview.

A good friend of mine, Arthur R. Pell, once wrote that an interview has four major purposes: to get information, to evaluate the applicant, to give information, and to make a friend.[1] In many interviews one or two of these purposes are satisfied while the rest remain uncovered.

If you are going to make an intelligent placement decision, you must obtain maximum information from the applicant. This requires sensitive listening skills. The ratio of interviewer talking to interviewer listening is critical. In the average 45-minute interview, the applicant should talk more than half the time. Since it is equally important for the applicant to judge you and your firm or institution, it is essential that the applicant receive basic information about the job, the institution, and career opportunities.

As important as eliciting and giving information is the evaluation process. It is not uncommon for the supervisor's personal bias to intrude upon the effective evaluation of a candidate. Biases can be favorable or unfavorable. We often like certain things about people and, therefore, are impressed when an applicant shows one of those favorable traits. Some of us are impressed by the way an applicant dresses or combs his or her hair. Still others are sensitive to speech mannerisms. (How often have you been impressed by someone with an English accent?)

Some interviewers rely on pseudoscience and mythology. Too many interviewers believe they can detect "the criminal type," or harbor prejudices against fat people (they are jovial or they are lethargic!), or against redheads (they are always unintelligent!). The "natural" judges of character are as unreliable as the myths about such judgments. Of course, appearance is not a reliable predictor of personality traits.

The intrusion of personal bias and pseudoscience has produced an alarming proportion of "quick sets." Very often interviewers allow their initial impression of a candidate to influence their final decision. One researcher found that most personnel interviewers made their decisions after just four minutes of a fifteen-minute interview.[2] This is unfortunate because very often an initial impression is positively or negatively affected by intensive exploration with the candidate over a much longer period. I am reminded of the silent screen star whose good looks and swashbuckling manner produced an aura of masculinity, but whose soprano voice doomed his career when talking movies were introduced. The opposite is often true as well. An individual who may not look the part may very well be just the person for the job.

Some supervisors are reluctant to vary their approach to interviews. Stereotyping interviews—that is, falling into a comfortable routine— often is nonproductive because of the different types of people who present themselves for interviews. The successful interviewer is flexible in approach and tries to be aware of the applicant's personality and needs.

According to Pell one purpose of the interview is to "make a friend." Keep in mind that every unsuccessful applicant is often a member of the community served by your institution. Impressions made in the interview situation are lasting ones. Common courtesy, a dignified approach, and a sympathetic rejection will be remembered even though the job was not offered. For the applicant who is successful, first impressions of the institution— usually obtained in the initial interview— are brought into the work area and can aid in developing an efficient and dedicated employee. When you interview an applicant for employment, you are functioning as a public relations arm of the institution. A dignified interview, with ample opportunity for the applicant to present his or her credentials, will be of immeasurable encouragement to the new employee in a new institution.

THE FIVE STAGES OF THE INTERVIEW

The Warm-Up Stage

It is essential that you establish rapport with the candidate who is often apprehensive about the interview. Diving into a cold pool can be quite a shock; it is often best to wade into cold water. Remember this when the applicant comes in and identifies himself or herself to you. Most applicants are tense; tension will affect the productivity of the interview. It is essential that you invest the time to put the applicant at ease.

This can be accomplished in many ways. Make an effort to establish a proper setting for the interview. If you seem harried and give the impression that this interview is a necessary evil, then the applicant will be defensive and often unresponsive. Talk about the weather; talk about transportation— ask if the applicant found it easy to get to the institution or found your office without difficulty. Don't have the applicant sit and wait while you look over the application blank; review the form before the applicant comes into the room. Don't open the interview with a caustic or insensitive question.

When someone asks me how long the warm-up period should take, I often reply, "As long as it will take to put the applicant at ease and in a nondefensive frame of mind." Sometimes you may be able to base your warm-up question on an item that appears in the application blank. Move on to the next stage when the applicant is talking and freely exchanging information with you.

The Applicant Talking Stage

Once again refer to the application blank and ask an open-ended question. Questions that can be answered with a simple "yes" or "no" are not effective. "I see that you worked at Metropolitan General Hospital for three years. Can you tell me about your job and what you did there?"

Now is the crucial test— can you keep your mouth shut? The idea is to let the applicant talk; let the applicant set the pace. The extent to which you may have to ask questions and guide the interview will depend entirely on the applicant. There will be enormous pressure on you to keep the conversation flowing, and there will be the problem almost all inexperienced interviewers face— handling periods of silence. I strongly advise you to resist the temptation to step into the breech. The applicant will eventually move on, and very often reveal critical points about his or her character or experiences.

The Questioning Stage

Remember, there is no set combination of questions that will be satisfactory for every interview. Pell gives us the most helpful review of the types of questions applicable in most situations.

1. *"W" questions:* The "W" questions—"what?" "when?" "where?" "who?" and "why?"—coupled with "how?" are useful in most interviewing situations.

2. *Leading questions:* Too often these questions move the applicant to give the answer that he or she thinks the interviewer wants. Leading questions should be discouraged, but they may be used to control the interview or to stop digressions.

3. *Probing questions:* These are incisive and specific questions used to obtain more detail about a specific activity or area. When a probing question is asked, the interviewer should be quite familiar with the area being examined.

4. *"Yes"-"No" questions:* This type of question may be used sparingly. A yes-no question cannot stand alone, since the form of the question does not give the applicant the opportunity to expand the answer.

5. *Situational questions:* The interviewer poses hypothetical problems and encourages the applicant to answer. In so doing, the applicant reveals knowledge and understanding of a subject. This type of question can be effective if the hypothetical problem is close to reality.

6. *Clarification and reflection questions:* This type of questioning essentially "mirrors" the interviewee's answers. It is used to get a fuller understanding of a question previously answered.[3]

It is a good idea to prepare your questions in advance of the interview. It is nonproductive to overload the applicant with a series of rapid-fire questions so that the interviewee is forced to remember the three or four questions posed in succession. Again, remember that the successful interviewer speaks far less than the applicant, even when giving information about the job. This often gives the applicant an opportunity to ask questions and make comments that can be evaluated.

It is most helpful in the questioning stage to give the applicant the impression you are genuinely interested in his or her background. This can be accomplished by putting yourself in the applicant's position. Remember the strain of an interview when you were on the other side of the table? Beware of being argumentative in this "drawing out" stage. If you disagree with an answer, it is not essential for you to correct the applicant or argue. If you feel that the applicant is holding back information, not telling the complete truth, it may be best to avoid a confrontation and assume a sympathetic posture. This can result in finally arriving at the complete and true story.

Employer Informational Stage

Supervisors often forget that there are two decisions to be made in an interview. First is the supervisor's decision as to the match: Does the applicant fit the job? Should an offer be made? The second decision is one that falls to the applicant: Do I want to work for this institution?

It is essential that the supervisor provide the applicant with all pertinent information concerning the job itself and the institution in general. Tell the applicant the what, why, how, and when of the job, and answer any questions. This can be a most revealing part of the interview, since the applicant's questions often are indicative of his or her value system.

Too often this part of the interview is rushed or underrated. Too many times I have heard newly hired employees state that the job to which they are assigned is quite different from the job explained to them in the interview.

A most helpful tool in the informational stage of the interview is a job description and, if one is available, a job specification. The job description often contains a job summary section that gives the applicant (and most important, the interviewer) an overall concept of the purpose, nature, and extent of the task performed. It also shows how the job differs generally from others in the organization. The job specification is also invaluable, as it contains the personal requirements, necessary skills, and the physical demands of the job. The job specification form commonly includes the requirements for education, experience, initiative, and ingenuity. Physical demands, working demands, and unavoidable hazards are outlined. A job description and a job specification are indispensable to the interview and placement process.

It is incorrect to assume that a supervisor and a subordinate are in fair agreement about the nature of the subordinate's job when they are discussing some plan or decision affecting the subordinate's work. A study conducted on superior-subordinate communications in management concluded that:

> ... if a single answer can be drawn from the detailed research study (presented in the report) into superior-subordinate communication on the managerial level in business, it is this: If one is speaking of the subordinate's specific job—his duties, the re-

quirements he must fulfill in order to do his job well, his intelligent anticipation of future changes in his work, and the obstacles which prevent him from doing as good a job as possible—the answer is that he and his boss do not agree or differ more than they agree in almost every area.[4]

This kind of misunderstanding too often starts at the original placement phase. Applicants should be absolutely certain about the duties and requirements of the job for which they are being interviewed; this is the responsibility of the immediate supervisor who will make the placement choice.

In either this stage or the previous one, there are questions that can be extremely helpful in revealing the applicant's lifestyle, personal philosophy, and general character. Here are some sample questions in that area:

1. What books have you read over the last six months?

2. Looking back over the last several years, what is the most important way in which you have changed in that time?

3. Where do you want to be— as far as your work is concerned— in the next three years, five years, ten years?

4. What are some of the things you do when you are not working— your hobbies and outside interests?

The Wind-Up Stage

To know when and how to conclude an interview comes with experience. The inexperienced supervisor will often end an interview abruptly and many times on a less than positive note. Be careful not to abort an interview based on a very quick, surface evaluation of the applicant. It may well be that you will cut down the amount of time spent in the interview because it is obvious that the individual being interviewed is not up to the standards of the job. It has been my experience over many years of interviewing at all levels that intuition and initial feelings are not the best guides for proper placement. Sometimes an applicant takes a long time to warm up, and initial negative vibrations change much later in the interview. It is your duty to give the applicant a fair chance to reveal a *complete* picture of his or her qualifications, motivations, and aspirations. It is also important that you not let the interview drag on, that you close at the right time, that you end on a positive note, and that you leave the applicant with a positive impression of your institution.

DOs AND DON'Ts IN JOB INTERVIEWING

At this juncture it is helpful to list those factors that make an interview successful and productive and those that are counterproductive to sound placement.

1. Do not stereotype your interview.

2. Do not allow the interview to assume the character of a comfortable routine.

3. Do not fall back on selecting only those candidates who show previous experience similar to that of the job in question.

4. Do not overhire. That is, do not select someone whose ability far exceeds that required by the job.

5. Do not be overly formal. Getting the applicant to relax is essential for a productive interview.

6. Do not give advice to the applicant. This is a preemployment stage and your only responsibility is to *select* a candidate appropriate for the position.

7. Do not be impatient. Let the interview run as long as necessary to develop a proper evaluation of the candidate.

8. Do maintain control over the interview. If the conversation is wandering, bring the applicant back on the track. If his or her responses are too general, ask for relevant details.

9. Do familiarize yourself with the job specification and job qualifications.

10. Do prepare in advance for the interview, permitting enough time and enough privacy.

11. Do not speak more than the applicant does. A good gauge would be to limit your talking to one-third of the time. (Anything less than half of the time will do).

12. Do leave the applicant with a favorable impression of the institution.

13. Do not set inappropriate standards for the job—either too high or too low.

14. Do not judge the applicant by one favorable or unfavorable attribute. (The "halo" effect is detrimental to overall evaluation.)

15. Do know your biases and do not let them interfere with the evaluation process.

16. Do not reach a conclusion *before* the interview has started (this happens more often than we are willing to admit) or before the interview has been completed.

17. Do not reveal by either word or expression that you are critical of the applicant's responses.

18. Do not interrupt the applicant unless he or she is wandering or not specific.

19. Do review, in advance of the interview, the application blank and any personnel tests or references.

In any list of "don'ts" it can be helpful to review some of the mistakes that inexperienced interviewers make. Dr. Arthur Witkin, an industrial psychologist, presents six classic mistakes.

1. The interviewer "telegraphs" the answer expected on each question. This results in a yes-no response.

2. The interviewer tries to scare or intimidate the applicant, by setting up traps. Very little will be revealed about the applicant's real self since he or she is too busy defending to reveal anything.

3. The interviewer does all the telling—about the company, about the job, about his or her own work, about his or her own family. The interviewer is in love with the sound of his or her own voice.

4. The interviewer is so busy writing down every word the applicant utters that there is no time for listening, looking, and reacting. After the interview, the interviewer really doesn't know what kind of person the applicant is.

5. The interviewer is busy filling out "an application blank." The interview consists of getting references, statistics, salaries, dates.

6. The interviewer believes in intuition and is a "stargazer." He or she sees qualities in the applicant that no one else is able to see.[5]

THE SCREENING INTERVIEW

In situations where a great number of applicants apply, it is important to conduct a screening of the candidates as quickly as possible to save time for the supervisor and the applicants. In many instances the personnel department is responsible for the preliminary screening, but there may be occasions when this is the supervisor's responsibility. Here, briefly, are the objectives of the screening interview:

1. to determine whether the job applicant is *generally* qualified for a specific job opening,

2. to determine whether the job applicant is qualified for other present or future openings in the department or in the institution, and

3. to make a favorable impression on the job applicant. (It is essential to create a favorable public relations impact on all applicants who contact the institution for a job.)

The screening interview is designed to limit the number of applicants given a placement interview. While recruitment is a magnet— its prime objective is to attract as many candidates as possible— screening is more a sieve to let through only those candidates who might well qualify for the job. It is important that the applicant feel his or her candidacy has been reasonably considered. Therefore, although the screening interview is short, it should not be uncomfortably rushed.

One of the best ways to expedite the screening interview is to identify those elements in the candidate's qualifications most crucial in determining his or her possible suitability for the job. For example, the nature of the position may require the employee to work overtime or to work unusual hours. If the interviewer spends thirty minutes determining the applicant's technical knowledge and experience and then finds out that he or she is unwilling to work the required hours, valuable time has been wasted. It is important to recognize that the screening interview is merely an opportunity to determine in a rather *general* way whether or not the applicant is qualified for the job opening. Intensive consideration of technical qualifications and personality should be left for the latter stages of the interview or for the placement interview. The primary objective of the *screening* interview is to put the candidate at ease and determine as rapidly as possible if he or she meets the basic requirements. The purpose of the *placement* interview is to determine specifically and in depth whether the applicant's work habits, attitudes, and personality are compatible with the job and with the institution.

AFFIRMATIVE ACTION

You and the applicant are not alone in the employment interview; sitting in are unseen but still powerful participants— the federal government and its partner, the state government. Various legislation affects the employment interview and, more importantly, circumscribes behavior that may have been possible prior to the enactment of such legislation.

It is now firmly established, if not finally interpreted, that employers must make a special effort to hire individuals who are deemed to be in a *protected class*. The law defines a protected class as one of several minorities that have been subjected to discrimination in hiring and promotion in past years: blacks, Spanish-surnamed Americans, Asian Americans, American Indians, and women. Special emphasis is placed on the several areas of the employment process where *rejection* is possible. These sensitive areas are:

1. in the general prescreening of applicants through replies to ads, walk-in candidates, and any other system of applying for a job;

2. in the most controversial arena of testing;

3. in the two forms of selection interviews—screening and placement;

4. in any checks—such as security checks, reference checks, or physical examinations—which may result in rejection.

Affirmative action is mandated by federal, state, and local laws in addition to presidential executive orders and court decisions. It would be most helpful if the supervisor were provided with the operative legislation in the area of equal employment opportunity, such as:

1. Title VII of the Civil Rights Act of 1964, as amended by the Equal Employment Opportunity Act of 1972. Chances are great that your institution is covered by this act since it applies to organizations engaged in interstate commerce, employing 15 or more persons; all educational institutions, public and private; state and local governments; public and private employment agencies; labor unions with 15 or more members; and joint labor-management committees for apprenticeship and training.

2. Executive Order 11246, as amended by Executive Order 11375. This affects federal contractors and subcontractors with 50 or more employees and contracts of $50,000 or more. It requires an employer to have an approved affirmative action program on file with the Office of Federal Contract Compliance Programs.

3. The Equal Pay Act of 1963 as amended by the Education Amendments of 1972 (Section 6(d) of the Fair Labor Standards Act). This specifically requires that organizations pay their female employees, both those exempt and nonexempt from the Fair Labor Standards Act, the same salary that their male employees receive for doing basically similar work.

4. The Age Discrimination and Employment Act of 1967, as amended in 1978 specifically prohibits discrimination against persons between the ages of 40 and 70.

5. The Rehabilitation Act of 1973, as amended in 1974. Again the employer is required to maintain an affirmative action program, in this case ensuring the hiring and promotion of qualified handicapped people.

6. The Vietnam Era Veterans Readjustment Act of 1974. This extends the protection of affirmative action on behalf of disabled veterans and veterans of the Vietnam era by contractors holding federal contracts of $10,000 or more.

7. Your state may well have passed legislation modeled on Title VII. You should become familiar with the State Equal Employment Opportunity Acts.

Health care organizations have been the subject of court action in the area of equal pay for men and women. In the past several years a federal district court ruled that an institution had violated the Equal Pay Act by paying its male attendants 30¢ an hour more than its female nursing aides;[6] another court decided that there was no distinction between the work performed by hospital male orderlies and female aides, and that the higher wages paid to the male orderlies were illegal under the Equal Pay Act;[7] another court declared that the job duties in a hospital for male orderlies and female nursing aides did not differ and that the higher pay scales for orderlies was unjustified;[8] in another case, California's Fair Employment Practice Commission ruled that a hospital discriminated against a minority worker, an American Indian, when she was not rehired as a laundry worker after a leave of absence, although the hospital then employed other people for similar laundry jobs.[9]

As a supervisor doing the actual hiring, you may find yourself on the "hot seat" because of recent court decisions and settlements involving reverse discrimination. In one hospital a suit was brought by a male private duty nurse against the hospital for not referring him for duty with female patients. The court decided that the hospital was unfairly discriminating against the male nurse and ordered administration to reach a satisfactory agreement with the nurse regarding future assignment policy.[10]

Members of groups not included in the protected classes listed under various acts are beginning to test the morality of affirmative action and question systems of quotas for protected classes. As a supervisor you must be up-to-date on the requirements of affirmative action laws. If your institution has an affirmative action plan, review it—specifically the hiring and promotion goals—to identify areas of underutilization of protected classes.

MAKING THE RIGHT CHOICE

The final decision to hire or not hire a particular candidate should be based upon a *battery of assessments*. It helps to work from a planned checklist of interviewing findings, covering:

1. *Previous experience:* Although it may not be necessary for the applicant to have exactly the same experience outlined in the job description, you should consider similar job duties, similar working conditions, and same degree of supervision exercised and/or received on previous jobs.

2. *Education and training:* You should review the candidate's formal education, major fields of study, and specialized training.

3. *Manner and appearance:* Consider general appearance, speech, nervous mannerisms, self-confidence, and aggressiveness.

4. *Emotional stability and maturity:* Consider friction with former supervisors, relationships with peers, reasons for leaving previous jobs, and job stability. Consider sense of responsibility and attitude toward work and toward family.

Still another checklist separates interviewing impressions into two areas:

1. *Personality factors:* You should determine what the applicant liked best and least about his or her previous job. The answer may reveal attitudes or patterns of behavior that may be useful in evaluating the applicant's suitability for the present opening. Perhaps the candidate will indicate a preference for jobs that are closely supervised or those that require independent action. Does the applicant want a job that does not demand too much or one that is routinized? Your questions should allow the applicant to reveal plans for the future. Does he or she see this job opening as temporary or as a career commitment? Did the applicant understand each question and reply directly to the point? Was the applicant uncommunicative or were replies responsive? Was the applicant spontaneous or more thoughtful in response to questions? Most important is consistency— was there internal agreement between the various answers and descriptions given by the candidate?

2. *Nonpersonality areas:* The candidate's educational background is important to any evaluation. Is the applicant's education adequate for the position, more than adequate, or less than adequate? Will the applicant need specific training? References should be reviewed before final evaluation. References completed by the applicant's former

direct supervisors are usually the best and most accurate. It may be possible to obtain such references by telephone checks planned in advance and handled by your personnel department. Specific attention should be directed toward verifying the job held by the applicant, the job duties described by the applicant, and the reasons for leaving that job. Ask former employers whether they would rehire the applicant. In general, two specific areas should be checked out through references:

   a. the applicant's performance, and
   b. the applicant's work habits, personal habits, and ability to get along with supervisors, subordinates, and fellow workers.

Pell has some cogent recommendations on evaluating an applicant and making an offer. He lists areas of "do" and areas of "do not."

"*Do*"—Be specific in letters requesting references; use the telephone where possible in checking references; plan the reference interview in advance; understand the advantages and limitations of using outside investigative agencies; have realistic physical and medical standards for each position; make the job offer in person or by telephone; confirm the offer by letter.

"*Do not*"—Pay much attention to letters of reference carried by applicants; forget to ask a former employer why an applicant left his job; forget to ask if the company would rehire the applicant; make the job offer before reference reports are completed; accept a bad reference without question. (The reference may be based on a personal dislike of the applicant by someone in the company. Check it with other sources if it does not appear consistent with all other factors.)[11]

Here is still another breakdown of the essential factors that make the interview effective and more scientific:

1. Limit the interview to areas that cannot be measured by other methods. Tests, the application blank, and reference checks augment the interview. Remember that the interview is a public relations opportunity where you are marketing the worth of your institution.
2. Train yourself in interviewing techniques. Ask your personnel department to develop an interview training seminar, or attend a seminar given by a local college or hospital or home association.
3. The prime purpose of the interview is to ascertain whether the applicant would fit in with your work group and be content with the work, and whether the applicant has the qualifications to do the assigned duties.

4. In the best selection programs the interview will only be one of a number of selection methods used.

5. In order to be successful, the interviewer should have complete knowledge of job requirements, working conditions, and supervisory preferences before beginning the interview.[12]

Key Points for the Interviewing Process

Finally review this list of reminders when evaluating your interviewing technique.

1. Become knowledgeable about affirmative action regulations and laws.

2. To match the person to the job, know in advance what the job is: review the job description, the job specifications, and profiles of employees who have successfully held similar jobs.

3. Assemble all the information about the candidate before you start the interview. Use the application blank, the resume (if available), references, and other preinterview information.

4. Plan the interview in advance. Don't stereotype the interview, but in general remember to establish rapport and communicate to the applicant complete information on job content and institutional policy.

5. Permit time for an exchange of information, including the answering of all questions.

6. Keep in mind that there are two decisions in every interview: Your decision to hire or not hire the candidate, and the candidate's decision to accept or not accept the position.

7. Look for potential. Don't be misled by the "myth of previous experience." Look for transferable experience.

8. Never forget that the candidate is under unusual stress. Do not minimize this tension, as it can affect the quality of the interview.

9. Accept the fact that you are a representative of the institution and perform a public relations function in all interviews. There is an opportunity to make friends even though you cannot make offers.

NOTES

1. Arthur R. Pell, *Recruiting and Selecting Personnel* (New York: Simon and Schuster, 1969), p. 102.

2. E. C. Webster, *Decision-Making in the Employment Interview* (Montreal: Industrial Relations Center, McGill University, 1964), pp. 13-14.

3. Pell, *op. cit.,* pp. 105-106.

4. N. R. S. Maier et al. *Superior-Subordinate Communications in Management, Report No. 52* (New York: American Management Association, 1961), p. 9.

5. Arthur Witkin, *Which Interviewer Are You?* (New York: Personnel Psychology Center of New York), pamphlet.

6. Hodgson v. G. W. Hubbard Hospital of Meharry Medical College, 351 F. Supp. 1295 (D.C., Md., Tenn., 1971).

7. Hodgson v. Brookhaven General Hospital, 470 F. 2d 729 (C.A. 5, 1972).

8. Brennan v. Prince William Hospital Corporation, 503 F. 2d 282 (C.A. 4, 1974).

9. Northern Inyo Hospital v. Fair Employment Practice Commission, 38 Cal. App. 3d 14 (1974).

10. Sibley Memorial Hospital v. V. Wilson, 488 F. 2d 1338 (C.A. D.C., 1973)

11. Pell, *op. cit.,* pp. 150-151.

12. Milton M. Mandell, *Recruiting and Selecting Office Employees, Research Report No. 27* (New York: American Management Association, 1956), p. 73.

Chapter 3

How To Avoid the High Cost of Turnover: Getting the New Employee Started

There is general agreement among management experts that a large proportion of turnover occurs with new employees, especially during the first month. Supervisors play a critical role in getting the new worker started on a job and often must act as vocational guidance specialists. The first days on a new job can make the difference between a productive, efficient employee and one who may soon become dissatisfied and leave.

Angelo Patri, a specialist in child development, was asked by a mother, "When should I begin teaching my six-month-old son the way to behave?" "Madam," he replied, "you are already six months too late!" The first few days and few weeks on the job are difficult ones for the employee and for the supervisor. Both must make an adjustment. The supervisor has the responsibility for balancing the employee's abilities and personality against the requirements of the job. The prompt integration of the new employee into the work force can yield optimum efficiency in minimum time. The cost of turnover is not a small one. When one considers the time, effort, and salaries expended in recruiting, interviewing, checking references, processing and training new employees, it is easy to understand the urgent need to reduce turnover during the probationary period.

Placement refers to the assignment of new employees to specific jobs and their melding into the larger work teams; *induction* is the process by which placement is made effective. If I were asked, "When should I start inducting and orienting my employees?", the answer would be "You are already days, weeks or months too late." Induction and orientation begin on the very first day of employment.

THE INDUCTION AND ORIENTATION PROGRAM

Objectives

For an induction and orientation program to succeed, its objectives must be clearly stated and communicated to all supervisors and employees. There are four general objectives of a successful induction and orientation program:

1. *To reinforce the employee's confidence in his ability to cope with a new work assignment.* Despite the fact that applicants often present a positive view of their ability to handle the job opening, on the first day of work, the employee is faced with a myriad of doubts. Most individuals fear criticism. Even when criticism is judiciously applied, it serves as a threat to self-confidence, and at no time is there a greater need to feel worthy than that first day on a new job.

First impressions remain with an employee for many years. He or she will approach the new assignment with some apprehension, with many predetermined attitudes carried over from home, school, church, and previous jobs, and certainly with the sense of not belonging. These new employees are not all the same—they react differently to criticism; some are aggressive; some are shy; some get angry quickly; some are introspective. They think differently; their ability to "catch on" differs. It is the supervisor's task to understand these basic differences among people and alter the induction and orientation program to meet different needs.

Differences notwithstanding, most new employees want to be a member of a purposeful group; they want to be accepted into the work team as quickly as possible. Some of them may have done a similar job in other institutions—"but not quite the way you do it here." Once people do a job in a certain way, they form habits and become resistant to change. In order to change habits, you must change attitudes. Offer a complete explanation of "why" things are done in a certain way. Therefore, another objective of the induction and orientation program is. . .

2. *To communicate complete and detailed conditions of the person's employment.* Although this should have been covered in the placement interview, the applicant may have been under tremendous pressure during that interview and did not absorb all that you and the personnel interviewers communicated. Thus, there is a need for further communication at a more receptive time—after placement, during the induction period. An employee who knows what must be done, why it

must be done in the prescribed way, and understands why his or her contribution is important to the total institution is likely to be more efficient and loyal.

3. *To inform the person of the rules and regulations surrounding employment.* In the first day or week of employment, the new employee has not formed any strong opinions and is far more receptive to an explanation of the rules and regulations of the institution, the "laws of the shop." The basic purpose of induction is to help employees become adjusted to their role as members of the work team. In addition to understanding the team's objectives and how they are attained, the new employee must know what constitutes acceptable behavior for the work team.

4. *To instill in the employee a feeling of pride in the institution.* Although it is true that the modern work area and work system is routinized, and that standardized techniques have robbed the worker of much of the emotional reward and sense of ownership that early craftsmen felt, it is equally true that with proper opportunity and encouragement, employees will gain a sense of the purpose of their work at whatever level it may be. Everyone's job can be "important" if there is an understanding of the interrelationship and interdependence of various jobs in the work team. It is difficult for individuals today to find satisfaction in their work, as in the days of the handicraft system. Special attention must be directed to the employee's desire to gain satisfaction from work and take pride in the "end product."

Policy

The supervisor must develop in the new employee an understanding of the ultimate goals of the institution and how the new employee contributes to the success of the these goals—patient care, teaching, or research.

As a supervisor you should be aware of your institution's policy—a clear statement of philosophy regarding the institution's approach to employees. Here are some key statements as to that commitment:

1. Human resources are our most precious asset and require both our understanding and our empathy.

2. Each new employee who joins the institution must be convinced that he or she is welcomed and needed.

3. All information necessary to acquaint the new employee with the job, the institution, and his or her fellow employees must be communicated at the very onset of employment.

4. The ultimate objectives of the institution and the role the new employees play in attaining these goals must be communicated. This communication does not end with the completion of the probationary period.

5. Induction is the first-line supervisor's responsibility. It is an ongoing process and may well make the difference between average, below average, or exceptional performance.

THE SUPERVISOR'S RESPONSIBILITY FOR EMPLOYEE ORIENTATION

There are several areas of responsibility that fall to the supervisor in the induction of a new employee into a department:

1. the establishment of a cordial and positive atmosphere;
2. the communication of orientation and training programs to the new employee;
3. the communication of the organizational structure of the department and specifically, how the department functions in relation to the rest of the institution;
4. the review of the job description and job specifications;
5. the introduction of a new employee to fellow workers;
6. a tour of the department, the work area and the institution;
7. communication of the rules and regulations of the institution and an explanation of the benefit programs available to the new employee;
8. the assignment of the new employee to a "sponsor." (For further details, see page 42); and
9. an evaluation program which follows up periodically on the new employee's progress.

These responsibilities can be incorporated in a specific induction program designed to meet the following overall objectives:

1. Make the new employee feel at ease with the institution, the new job, and new associates; give the new employee a proper first impression that will be positive and lasting.

2. Assist the new employee in understanding the total function of the institution; relate the ultimate function of the institution to the new employee's job.

3. Assist the new employee in understanding completely the conditions of employment and rules and regulations of the institution.

4. Assist the new employee in knowing and understanding the employee benefits and services available.[1]

STAFF AND LINE INDUCTION

The two main steps of an orientation program are (1) staff induction—usually performed by the personnel department and (2) line induction—always performed by the first-line supervisor.

Let us look first at the personnel department's responsibility. Induction starts at the hiring process. The first step in the hiring process is the interview, which may be viewed as the preemployment phase of induction. The physical setting of the personnel department is an important factor in creating a favorable first impression. The next link in the induction process is the personnel interviewer. It is the responsibility of the employment interviewer to ensure that every prospective employee is given all the information necessary to understand the demands of the job, the rewards of the job, and to acquaint themselves with the working environment. The staff orientation phase is continued in the final placement interview conducted by the supervisor. The supervisor's responsibility does not end with the placement interview, however. The employee's first day in the new department is a difficult one and should be a day of linkage between good staff induction and good line induction.

Line induction is the responsibility of the first-line supervisor and is not made unnecessary by the supervisor's role in the interviewing process. The supervisor must introduce a new employee to fellow workers. Although it is the first-line supervisor's primary responsibility, it can be delegated to specialists. Let us look at some of the techniques to consider in fulfilling the institution's obligation for proper induction:

1. *Notice of employment in writing with complete details.* Every new employee should receive in advance of reporting to work a written statement of the actual job offer. This statement should include the title of the position, a brief description of the position, the supervisor's name, the pay rate, and the reporting time and place. The supervisor is vital to the induction procedure and, therefore, the new employee should be directed to report to the office of the immediate supervisor. It is the supervisor's responsibility to escort the new employee to the work area and introduce him or her to fellow workers.

2. *Institutional tours.* Many successful induction programs feature institutional tours to key areas. This gives the new employee a broader

sense of the purpose of the organization and an opportunity to see areas that may be off-limits during subsequent employment with the institution.

3. *Employee handbooks.* Almost all successful induction programs include the distribution of an employee handbook. These handbooks contain a statement of policy, conditions of employment, obligations, and benefits. The purpose of an employee handbook is to provide the new employee with a complete overview on the institution's personnel administration so that policies and procedures approved by the institution's board are clearly understood. The handbook, therefore, is a natural offshoot of the personnel policy and procedure manual. Most good employee handbooks start off with a section on "getting started" which details the organization's selection policy, deals with proper induction of new employees, and explains the probationary period. A summary of the obligation of employees is included in a separate section and is a concomitant to the benefits and opportunities available to the employee. Employee manuals or handbooks are often illustrated and should attempt to present in a readable, informal, and understandable fashion information necessary to assist the new employee in acclimating to the new organization.

4. *A sponsorship or "buddy" system.* Sponsorship programs have found many adherents throughout the country. A senior employee is selected to be the "buddy" of a new employee and ease adjustment to the new work situation. The sponsor talks with the newcomer, is a companion during rest periods, helps interpret rules and customs of the work area, and in general, attempts to make the new employee feel at ease in the new surroundings. (See Exhibit 1).

5. *Informational lectures and films.* These are used widely in induction programs. All recently hired employees are invited to an orientation session, usually scheduled in the first week of employment. Most successful programs have mandatory attendance requirements. A staff specialist from the training department usually chairs the conference and provides a detailed and, in many cases, illustrated lecture on the nature of the institution, its policies, employment practices, safety programs, and employee services. Specialists in those areas may be called upon to address the group and answer questions. A film may be shown. These films are usually obtainable from local or national hospital or home associations. However, it is possible to produce at low cost a film that deals with your institution's specialized situation.

WHAT THE NEW EMPLOYEE SHOULD LEARN
ON THE FIRST DAY OF WORK

Here are some of the things a new employee should learn the first day or certainly the first week on the job:

1. the routine of the job,
2. the functions and workings of other parts of the organization,
3. how to find one's way around the institution,
4. how this job fits into the larger picture,
5. what the privileges of a new employee are,
6. who one's associates and fellow workers are,
7. the history of the institution and how it services the community today,
8. how most employees are interdependent, and
9. what are the channels for exchanging ideas and information.

AN ALIEN IN THE NEW COUNTRY

Although many new employees have had experience in similar institutions, there will be some who must adjust to a completely foreign environment. A socializing process must take place to encourage good communication and behavioral patterns. Dubin offers the following explanation of the basic problems of orientation and induction.

> Orientation and indoctrination of a new member are essentially processes of acculturation. He has to learn ways of behaving, a set of standards and expectations, and a point of view and outlook largely foreign to him in their specific details, although he may be generally familiar with them in their broad outline. A great deal of the new employee's time may be spent during his early weeks and months of employment simply becoming adjusted to the organization.
>
> The adjustment process first involves becoming familiar with the language and its significant symbols that are used in the organization. In order for the new individual to understand how the organization operates and his role in it, he has to understand the language by which communication is carried out. Accordingly, at the initial stage of orientation and indoctrination, a great deal of attention is paid, both by the new member and by those who are teaching him, to learn a vocabulary and a set of

symbols that communicate significantly. In order to maximize understanding of what goes on, the new recruit has to become fairly familiar with the language of the organization.[2]

PROBATIONARY PERIOD

Most unionized institutions have labor contracts which contain provision for a probationary period. It permits the institution the unappealable right to terminate employment of new employees during either a 30-day, 60-day, 90-day or six-month probationary period. This period is a time for testing out the new employee. It is the supervisor's responsibility to evaluate the performance of a new employee so that a "go" or "no go" decision can be made before the expiration of the probationary period. It is critical to understand that once the employee completes the probationary period, seniority protection plays an essential role; indeed, there is a moral obligation for the institution to live within the due process mechanism of the labor contract or of personnel policies in the area of termination. Therefore, it is essential for the supervisor to follow up on new employees at various points during the probationary period. These are appropriate points at which to review with the employee his or her performance to date. It would be well for you to have a checklist of critical points in your evaluation of new employees. An employee who displays poor work habits during a probationary period is a bad risk for productive and efficient employment. It is the supervisor's responsibility to ensure that those added to the work force are likely to be satisfactory employees.

A REVIEW OF THE PRINCIPLES OF INDUCTION

The cost of sound and formal induction and orientation is small when compared to the high cost of employee turnover and inefficiency. These four principles of induction serve as the basis of a successful program and should neither be compromised nor neglected:

1. New members of a group or an institution must go through an extensive process of adjustment during which they must learn new rules and adapt old habits to the new group.

2. This adjustment can be facilitated by providing new employees with facts relating directly to their specific job and to employment in the institution as a whole.

3. As with all other important responsibilities of a health care institution, the responsibility for induction and orientation must be delegated clearly to a capable member or members of the management team. This responsibility must be understood. Although the line is ultimately responsible for induction, the staff may be delegated a substantial part of this burden.

4. The process of induction does not end after the first week or month of employment. Orientation is a long process, and in the final analysis it is the key link between good selection and good job performance.

Key Points in the Induction Process

1. Turnover is costly. The highest percentage of turnover occurs with new employees during the probationary period.

2. The supervisor has the main responsibility for induction and orientation of new employees. Although the personnel department, in its staff capacity, performs an essential function in the induction process, the supervisor is vital to successful assimilation and retention of employees.

3. Establishment of a cordial and positive atmosphere will make employees feel at home in an alien land. Mutual acceptance between the work group and the new employee is essential and must be expedited.

4. Good habits and bad habits are developed from the very start. The first few days and weeks on the job will be critical. Give the new employee a proper first impression that will be lasting and positive.

5. Ask the more responsible employees in your department to sponsor the new employees.

6. Indoctrination is not a short, one-step procedure. It requires follow up and attention over a protracted period of time. Don't lose interest; don't let the employee believe that you've lost interest. An early investment in this procedure will yield large dividends: and efficient employee, a long-term employee, a loyal employee.

NOTES

1. P. Ecker et al., *Handbook for Supervisors* (Englewood Cliffs, N.J.: Prentice-Hall, Inc., 1959), p. 131.

2. Robert Dubin, *The World of Work* (Englewood Cliffs, N.J.: Prentice-Hall, Inc., 1958), p. 337.

Exhibit 1   Supervisor (Sponsor) Induction Checklist

Employee Name _____ Date Reported _____
Department _____ Supervisor _____
Each step is designed to ease the adjustment of the new employee. Do not skip any point. Please check (x) off the steps as you cover them with the new employee. Forward this completed form to the Personnel Department.

- - - - - - - - - - - - - - - - - -

_____   *Welcome the employee*
Introduce yourself; put him or her at ease

_____   *Explain work schedule*
Communicate hours, days off, lunch hour, holidays, free days, and vacation

_____   *Tell him about the department*
What the department does; the importance of the work; how his or her job fits in

_____   *Pay*
Tell when pay day is, how much, chances for advancement, and review general dates for salary review

_____   *Rules and regulations*
Suggest the employee review the employee manual "All About Your Job," including rules and regulations

_____   *Illness or accident on the job*
Advise employee to go to health service or emergency room

_____   *Uniforms, lockers, parking, bathrooms, and rules of dress and cleanliness*
Explain, locate, and familiarize

_____   *Explain the job*
1. Prepare: Arouse interest, put at ease
2. Demonstrate: Tell, show, illustrate, ask
3. Try out: Have employee do; explain, correct errors
4. Follow up: Tell employee where to get help; check frequently

_____   *Show department and introduce to coworkers*
Introduce employee to responsible supervisor with whom he or she may deal

————————   *Have someone accompany new employee to lunch*

————————   *FOLLOW UP:* At end of week, check progress; review employee manual; encourage questions

- - - - - - - - - - - - - - - - -

The above induction steps have been covered with the employee.

_____   _____
Signature of Sponsor   Signature of Supervisor
(if not supervisor)

_____   _____
Date   Date

Chapter 4
How To Evaluate Performance

The classic studies in employee motivation point out the importance of full appreciation for a job well done. The average employee wants to "feel in on things"—know what is going on in the department and in the institution in general; how that affects his or her own job; how he or she is doing in the eyes of the supervisor.

One cannot discuss the need for appreciation without looking at the other side of the coin. Employees often express deep fear of criticism. No one likes to be told he or she is doing something improperly; no one likes to be chastised; few employees are willing to admit they are wrong if it appears to demean them in the eyes of their peers.

Performance appraisal is without a doubt one of the most complex and controversial areas of the supervisor-subordinate relationship. It seems not to matter what rank the employee holds in the organization—employees want to know where they have been, where they are now, and where they are going. They want to know what the institution and, more importantly, what their immediate supervisor expects of them. They want to know how well they have performed and how their performance was measured. If it is presented properly, they want to know which areas need improvement. Finally, they want to know how they can move ahead in the institution. On the other hand, it seems not to matter at which level an executive is in the institution—whether a first-line supervisor, a department head, or an assistant director: Almost all managers dislike and question the necessity to criticize a subordinate's work.

Many supervisors will say it is easier to say nothing. Often supervisors will comment, paradoxically, it is easier to terminate a subordinate's employment than do the distasteful work of improving his or her performance. Merrihue stated,

> The supervisor who obtains the best from his employees is the one who creates the best atmosphere or climate of approval within which his work group operates; he accomplishes this through the following methods: (1) he develops performance standards for his employees and sets them high to stretch the employees; (2) he measures performance against these standards, (3) he consistently commends above-par performance; (4) he always lets employees know when they have performed below par.[1]

Mayfield supports the Merrihue approach by insisting that every supervisor should appraise his or her subordinates periodically and communicate the results of this evaluation. He believes that the appraisal procedure and the progress interview are surprisingly effective and free from difficulties when used with reasonable judgment.[2]

But lest you think that all the experts are unequivocally in favor of performance evaluation, Odiorne writes, "I can see only mechanical policing methods to create the strictures of the deadening conformity. Individuality based on the capacity of each free man to express himself as a human being is not a value to be eradicated lightly, and it should be cherished."[3] He maintains we have wasted time and money on appraisal systems that could be better used for improving on-the-job training of managers to fulfill the basic task of leadership.

Does the appraisal program produce conformity? Is it the basis for remedial action? Is it the yardstick for the next salary increment? I believe that most critics of performance evaluation look at the mechanism too closely. We can be critical of the scales and ranking mechanisms, the list of personality traits, or the impossible rush toward the arena of empirical judgment. On the other hand, there is a side of appraisal programs that seems to recommend their use to all first-line supervisors: the system reinforces performance by a systematic assessment of observable work achievements rather than by assessment of personality traits. What we will discuss here is a tool for a *plan for progress,* not for conformity and not for criticism. We must accept the fact that most employees, if they understand what is expected of them and if they receive the necessary assistance, will improve their performance. They *can* agree with their immediate supervisor on the aims and goals of the department and the institution. In effect, this puts the ball in your court: the first-line supervisor must inspire improvement and must develop the plan by which individual workers can become more efficient. In the arena of performance evaluation half the battle is won when the employee understands your expectations, how well he or she is meeting those expectations, and where improvement is needed.

A work group tends to elicit an employee's loyalty to the extent that it satisfies the employee's needs and helps the employee achieve goals. A worker tends to feel committed to a decision or goal depending on the degree to which the worker has participated in determining that goal— and understands why the goal has been set.

Each group is able to improve its operation to the extent that it consciously examines its processes and their consequences and experiments with improved processes. This is called the "feedback mechanism," a process originally used with guided missiles to correct any flight deviations by feeding back into their control mechanisms course data collected by sensitive instruments. The first-line supervisor must set high standards for the group that are communicated to each individual employee. This "feedback mechanism" is intended to keep the work group "on course." Maybe this appears to be a concerted effort to obtain conformity, but it isn't so if subordinates and the first-line supervisor work together to develop that course in the first instance.

PURPOSE OF PERFORMANCE EVALUATION

The primary purpose of performance evaluation is the improvement of job performance by:

1. communicating specific standards to employees and gaining acceptance of those standards;
2. measuring the employee's performance against the agreed upon standards;
3. developing with the employee a plan of action to assist the employee in overcoming obstacles to development and in strengthening his or her capabilities;
4. encouraging reactions, facing and resolving differences, and reaching a mutual understanding of the implications of the review; and
5. offering constructive suggestions and tangible assistance to the employee working toward personal development.

Performance evaluation programs are directed toward increasing the employee's understanding of what is expected on the job; how these expectations are being met; and how performance can be improved. In addition, the performance evaluation program provides the manager with a means of rating the worker's performance on a more objective basis.

Finally, it permits the supervisor to identify employees qualified for positions of greater responsibility.

OBJECTIVES OF EMPLOYEE PERFORMANCE EVALUATION

The American Hospital Association says a sound employee appraisal program should have the following objectives:

1. Systematic analysis of *all* important aspects of an employee's performance, not just isolated incidents of behavior or outstanding examples of good and poor performance. Be warned of the halo effect in evaluating employees—that is, judging a worker's entire performance on the basis of a good or bad selected incident. This may be quite different from what we shall see if we look at the entire performance over a protracted period of time and not unfairly affected by one or two incidents.

2. Application of uniform standards or a common measuring stick that all supervisors can apply in a like manner to all employees. One of the problems in evaluation is the discrepancy between assessments made by an "easy going" supervisor as compared with a "tough taskmaster" supervisor. There should be general agreement as to the measuring mechanisms and this is one area that requires particular attention.

3. Reduction of guesswork, favoritism, and influence in the evaluation of employee performance. One of the sore spots in the supervisor-subordinate relationship is the playing of favorites. The standards used to evaluate one employee's performance should be the same as those applied to all other employees.

4. Collection of objective evidence of the relative merits of various employees to enable management to justify promotion, transfer, salary adjustment, training, and termination on an equitable basis throughout the institution. There is a need for specific facts as to the merits or faults of employees. Wherever possible, evaluation should be based upon data accumulated over a period of time.

5. Provision for a method of comparing personnel costs with actual employee performance on the job. This kind of comparison goes to the heart of employee performance evaluation—and measures employee efficiency related to the direct labor costs of running the department.

6. Development of an inventory of the skills and abilities of the work force to ensure proper placement of each employee and to prevent wasted manpower. Most employees welcome the opportunity to be

evaluated so that they may be placed at the right job and have full opportunity to make use of their capabilities. Performance evaluation programs can be used to develop an inventory of skills so that proper placement is indeed guaranteed and proper utilization is equally assured.

7. Provision of a statement of individual progress of each employee, with specific indications of areas needing improvement. Employees want to know exactly how well they are doing and, equally as important, how they can improve their performance against their supervisor's expectations and standards.

8. Provision of a system for giving employees recognition and reward in proportion to their performance on the job. This objective fulfills the number one need expressed by employees—recognition of a job well done and appropriate rewards in relationship to performance.

9. Provision of practical instruction for training supervisory and management personnel in the evaluation, direction, and development of personnel. This training is necessary for proper implementation of evaluation programs. Special attention should be directed to development of interviewing skills and a system for standardizing evaluations.

10. Organization of facts that can serve as a basis for agreement in labor-management negotiations—in effect, provision of a method for defining the "other things being equal" clause in union contracts. This objective underscores the use of performance evaluations for backing up decisions in the areas of promotion, transfers, and discipline.

TYPES OF RATING SYSTEMS

Performance evaluation forms seem to take as many shapes as the number of institutions using them. The best rating scale is the one acceptable to the supervisor and to the employees. Reaching agreement is not a simple task. Let us look at our options:

1. *Rating scales.* Scales are developed in a graphic or multiple-step format. The supervisor makes a choice of an appropriate rating along the scale; the choice is indicated by checking off either a number or a description on the scale. The description might be in terms of "below average," "average," and "above average." It may be expressed in numbers from zero to ten—ten being the highest; it may be expressed in letters commonly used in schools, "A," "B," "C," "D" and "F." In effect, the supervisor is rating the employee against an absolute standard and not against another employee. It is a simple method and,

therefore, the most popular. Rating is often done on various traits—such as ambition, character, cooperation, responsibility, attendance, and punctuality.

2. *Checklists.* Checklists work in a way similar to rating scales, but instead of using a quantitative measurement (numbers, letters), each trait is followed by descriptive statements that offer the rater an opportunity to select an appropriate description of the employee's job performance. For example, the trait "cooperation" could be rated as follows:

a. exceptional cooperation, goes out of his or her way to cooperate and coordinate his or her activities with others;

b. the employee is cooperative, works harmoniously with other people, and is willing to help out other departments;

c. the individual is not exceptionally cooperative until the need is great and occasionally indulges in obstructive arguments;

d. the individual is often difficult to deal with, thinks only of own department or unit, and is obstructive.

The supervisor then chooses among these four descriptions of the trait the statement that best fits his or her evaluation of the employee's performance. Checklists often provide a quantification so that a final score of overall performance might be ascertained. The basic difficulty with checklists is the problem of selecting individual descriptions for the various ratings of a specific trait. This is not an easy task, and very often supervisors complain about the poor choices available to them on a checklist. This problem can be overcome by obtaining the first-line supervisor's input in the design of the form.

3. *Employee comparison systems.* These do not require the use of an absolute standard as in rating scales and checklists. The supervisor is asked to compare the employee with other employees being evaluated. To refine the comparison, the rating is done on a factor-by-factor basis. This method is used widely in the military. Of course, such a system cannot be used to rate employees who have unique jobs. Many supervisors find this method forces them to make ratings and makes performance evaluation an easier process.

4. *Goal Setting.* This system of performance evaluation is widely used and often referred to as *management by objectives* (MBO). Here the worker is rated according to the degree to which he or she attains predetermined job goals. Goals or objectives are qualitative and/or quantitative targets which *you and the employee agree on in advance.* It is essential that employees understand and accept the criteria against

which their performance will be judged. The criticisms of traditional merit rating systems in performance evaluation programs are often satisfied by using a program built around management by objectives.

Beatty and Schneier have evaluated the potential advantages and disadvantages of performance appraisal methods and find that management by objectives is "very good to excellent" inasmuch as it measures contributions to the "organization/department objectives." Its accuracy and credibility are highly effective with employees who also rated it "good to very good" as to its feedback potential. Because of its job-relatedness, it provides problem-solving performance review, ending with a plan for performance improvement, thereby reducing the "ambiguity/anxiety" of raters regarding which standards of job performance are required and expected by the raters or organization.[4]

The MBO process includes the following steps:

a. formulation of objectives by top administration,
b. the development of realistic action plans for attainment of goals by subordinates;
c. the systematic monitoring and measuring of performance and achievement;
d. the taking of corrective actions necessary to achieve the plan objectives after receiving feedback of results.[5]

Peter F. Drucker was the first to use management by objectives as the basis for a complete management system. He believed that through self-control and the formulation of clearly defined objectives, individual supervisors could become more highly motivated. Although the system has been mainly applied to supervisory and managerial positions, it is indeed applicable to all strata of the institution. The key to a successful MBO system is a more personal orientation to the appraisal mechanism. In addition to the objectives set by the institution itself, attention must be directed to individual goals. In the final analysis the success of the MBO system depends on the degree of mutual agreement over desired objectives for a specific department or a specific employee.

PERFORMANCE EVALUATION INTERVIEW

The performance evaluation interview is an important procedure but often yields less than satisfactory results. The supervisor should identify clearly the primary objective of such interviews: to aid employees to understand for themselves where they have been and where they are going—specifically, where improvement is needed and how they will be aided in meeting the agreed-upon standards. Thus the performance evaluation interview is a vehicle for indicating appreciation or disappointment and provides an unusual opportunity to discuss a plan for self-improvement.

Three steps are central to performance evaluation. The first step is preparation—knowing what to discuss and planning how to discuss it. The second is feedback, and the last is follow-up. The purposes of an appraisal or feedback interview are:

1. letting employees know where they stand,
2. helping employees do a better job by clarifying what is expected of them,
3. planning developmental and growth opportunities,
4. strengthening the superior/subordinate working relationship by developing a mutual understanding of expectations, and
5. allowing subordinates to express themselves concerning performance-related issues.[6]

It is essential that the employee know well in advance that the interview is to take place. He or she should understand that participation is essential and that questions are encouraged. It is important that the interview be held in privacy, without interruptions. Enough time should be scheduled so that there is no pressure on either of the participants. The key to the interview is open communication. The objective is to set goals mutually agreed upon as a result of a review of past performances and future expectations.

HUMAN VALUES AT THE CORE OF THE EVALUATION PROCESS

As a supervisor you must be genuinely interested in the people who work for you. You can display your interest and effect positive results if you implement the following plans:

1. Get your people to see the end results of purposeful, consistent effort on their part as it relates to the advancement of their own career.
2. Provide them with goal-oriented job descriptions.
3. Utilize incentive programs that will have purpose and meaning to them.
4. Show them how they fit into institution goals. Give them deserved praise and meaningful recognition.

5. Give them opportunity to achieve. Achievement in itself is a great motivator.

6. Determine what their personal goals are and try to tie these in with the goals of the institution.

7. Help them organize and maintain the spirit of achievement by carefully planning and organizing efforts toward the attainment of meaningful results.

8. Help them set and achieve self-improvement goals.

9. Acknowledge in public their accomplishments to satisfy the key need for recognition and for feeling important.

10. Help them believe that they are accepted and approved by the institution and by their bosses.

11. Show them how and why they are doing useful work.

12. Tell them about their progress.

13. Listen with interest to their problems, their ideas, and their grievances.

14. Show them how they can meet their goals through the institution and by meritorious performance.

15. Never neglect them, ignore them, forget them.[7]

Many of these suggestions are at the heart of a sound performance evaluation program.

Key Points for Appraising the Performance of Employees

1. Performance evaluation must be based on clear, well-defined, and fully communicated expectations and goals.

2. The performance evaluation process offers an opportunity to discuss past successes and past deficiencies; but it offers as well an opportunity to plan, counsel, and coach future improvement.

3. People will be better motivated if they know precisely what is expected of them, if they have the opportunity to obtain assistance as needed, if they know exactly how their supervisor feels about their performance and, finally, if they receive appropriate recognition when it is deserved.

4. Supervisors who do a good job in communicating their evaluation of an employee's performance will encourage reactions, face up to and resolve differences, and reach mutual understanding of the implications of the review. The successful supervisor is able to communicate to employees who have performed below standard and in-

terested enough to commend those who have attained above-stand-
ard performance.

NOTES

1. Willard Z. Merrihue, *Managing by Communication* (New York: McGraw-Hill Book Company, 1960), p. 122.

2. Harold Mayfield, "In Defense of Performance Appraisal," *Harvard Business Review*, March-April, 1960, pp. 81-87.

3. George S. Odiorne, "What's Wrong with Appraisal Systems?", *Personnel Policies: Issues and Practices* (Columbus, Ohio: Charles E. Merrill Books, 1964), p. 79.

4. Richard W. Beatty and Craig Eric Schneier, *Personnel Administration and Experimental Skill Building Approach* (Reading, Mass.: Addison-Wesley Publishing Company, 1977), pp. 81-82.

5. Anthony P. Raia, *Managing by Objectives* (Glenview, Ill.: Scott, Foresman and Company, 1973), p. 11.

6. Robert I. Lazer and Walter S. Wikstrom, *Appraising Managerial Performance: Current Practices and Future Directions* (New York: The Conference Board, A Research Report, 1977), p. 30.

7. Addison C. Bennett, "Effective Management Centers on Human Values," *Hospitals, JAHA*, July 16, 1976, pp. 73-75.

Chapter 5

How To Communicate
for Change

If there is a single consistency in today's complex health care industry it is the move toward change. As a supervisor you must initiate changes at a faster rate than ever before. Changes touch the organizational structure, personnel policies, procedures, equipment, techniques, technologies, and in general, the way health care is delivered. The supervisor has a key role in the communications grid. No matter what the change may be, the average employee will be suspicious and often resistant. To the employee in your department, there is no such thing as an insignificant change. Change implies a move from the old, comfortable, and mastered way to an unknown and threatening way. The best way to introduce the subject of communicating for change is to explore the normal reaction to the announcement of change—resistance.

RESISTANCE TO CHANGE

Resistance is behavior intended to protect the employee or group of employees from the effects of real or imagined change. Resistance is protective and often defensive in nature, and arises from either a real or imagined threat to the security of the individual or group. It is associated with feelings that range from hostility and aggression to apathy and withdrawal. Not fully understanding how the change will affect him or her, the employee feels suspicious and threatened. There are several conditions under which employees tend to resist change:

1. When the nature of the change and its effects are not clearly communicated and understood by those affected. Yet, the communication

55

of full information is not in and of itself a guarantee of the elimination of resistance.

2. When they are not prepared for the change. It is disastrous for an institution to announce a critical change to employees who have not been forewarned.

3. When employees have not been consulted in advance regarding the necessity for change and have not been included in discussions of alternatives to unproductive procedures or methods.

4. When information is distorted, especially if employees have felt uncomfortable and threatened in past work situations. Employees have long memories. Present assurances do not easily eradicate past disappointments.

5. When the change is made on personal grounds, rather than because of impersonal requirements of the group or the institution.

6. When the change ignores established norms or customs of the group.

7. When excessive work pressure is involved in the change. Employees are ever alert to the possibility that change will result in additional work, unfair distribution of the workload, and speed up.

8. When the planning of change fails to consider in detail exactly how the change will be brought about. Poor planning will ensure a disaster.

9. When insufficient consideration is given to problems that are likely to arise and how to deal with them.

10. When there is fear of failure or when the change is seen as inadequate or ineptly managed.

11. When it is not obvious why the change is needed and what was wrong with the old way of doing things.

Once people do things in a certain way, they form habits. Change requires a gradual weaning from the old habits, an alteration of attitudes. Attitudes, for the most part, can only be changed by experience—not as the result of facts. Almost every attempt to introduce change sets up a countervailing force familiarly termed "resistance to change," initiated by the employee whose job security, habits, or relationships seem to be threatened. Such resistance takes the form of anxious queries, wild rumors of impending disaster, grievances, noncooperation, slow-downs, refusal to meet new goals, or subtle group behavior to discredit the new system.[1]

One observer questions resistance to change and sees it more as resentment or anxiety over the way change is introduced. Trying to convince someone of the advantages of the new method often sounds like criticism of the old—which the employee likes because it is familiar or even because he or she sponsored it originally. More than one supervisor has flatly rejected a machine by saying either in anger or in hurt that there is nothing wrong with the performance of the department. Sometimes a change is introduced in a way that appears to threaten established work habits and relationships; it never gets a chance to be accepted in its own right. Many a supervisor has made a new process turn out to be just as impractical as he or she predicted it would be.[2]

OVERCOMING RESISTANCE TO CHANGE

Recent studies indicate that supervisors can best initiate change when they:

1. Use resistance as a diagnostic symptom to get at its cause.

2. Use feedback, the release of feelings, and the blowing off of steam to air resistance, bring it out in the open.

3. Allow the groups involved to make some decisions, within defined limits, on how to implement the change and on how problems will be handled.

4. Build a trusting work climate. Get and give honest answers to questions that relate to policy and procedures.

5. Communicate, discuss, encourage feedback, and help people gather facts pointing to the need for change as related to their own problems and needs.

6. Use group norms and customs in planning and implementing change.

7. Use two-way communication to help those affected develop:

   a. their own understanding of the need for change,
   b. explicit awareness of how they feel about the change, and
   c. understanding of what can be done about their feelings.[3]

The supervisor's role in overcoming resistance to change starts with the key questions: What is my plan for communicating change? What is my plan for ameliorating the effect of the change on the personnel involved?

It is essential that the reasons for the change be communicated in detail. Don't mask these reasons; don't rationalize them. If change is introduced to reduce costs or increase productivity, state it out front. Each employee must understand the impact on his own particular job. Essential to the selling of change is the encouragement of an exchange of concerns and information including the setting up of conditions under which employees are assured their questions will be answered.

A simple plan is to hold a group meeting where reasons for and details of the change are explained. This can be followed up with smaller group meetings. In these latter meetings you as an immediate supervisor will explore problems and concerns with your subordinates and attempt to ameliorate any apprehension. This can be followed with written communication to all employees. Of course, supervisors must be trained in advance of the change.

THE SUPERVISOR AS A CHANGE AGENT

Good communication is essential to good employee relations. The supervisor who does not communicate properly will often have an unproductive group. Reliable information is at the heart of communication. If the supervisor is not "in" on things, how can he or she be an effective communicator? It is essential that the supervisor know what is going on within the institution, what others expect of him or her, and what is planned for the future.

A willingness to include supervisors in the planning stage is one hallmark of an effective organization. If the supervisor knows what is expected and why, he or she can be a more productive communicator. He or she must give meaning to policy and procedure changes in the day-to-day work arena. Employees are quick to understand when the supervisor is "mouthing" institutional policy rather than "backing" such policy.

A downward flow of formal communications is typical of most institutions. Too often certain levels of the management hierarchy are bypassed, leading to problems. The supervisor who is bypassed may feel that he or she is an unnecessary link in that chain and fall into a negative pattern of working against the organization. No supervisor can support what he or she does not understand or has not been consulted about.

Let us step back at this point and substitute for the term "supervisor" the word "employee." It is easy to see how the employee's lack of understanding and participation will result in counterproductive behavior.

PSYCHOLOGICAL PRINCIPLES OF COMMUNICATION

There are certain psychological principles of communication that operate in the supervisor-subordinate relationship.

1. Whenever two people or groups of people come together, communication goes on. It is patently clear that no one can prevent people from communicating when they are in contact with each other. It is only the direction, quantity, and effectiveness of communication that can be controlled.

2. In all communication listening is as important as talking. Communication is a complete and closed circle. Listening is essential to the communication process.

3. Ideas can be transferred directly from one person to another. Mental filters and perceived meaning often produce static in the communication process. To the listener total meaning is a mixture of intellectual and emotional associations. That is why communication experts have paid so much attention to body language: facial expressions, gestures, and inflections can make or break communications.

4. Words do not have meaning within themselves. All of us derive meaning from experience and, therefore, words have different meaning to different people.

5. Meanings, attitudes, beliefs, and expectancies once established tend to remain stable. Present meanings, attitudes, and expectancies tend to be unconsciously supported and reinforced.

6. Because of already established attitudes and expectancies, certain methods of communication and certain communicators may be rejected. There is no question that much of the rejection is emotional.[4]

FEEDBACK

Since it is difficult to convey meaning and the full meaning of any message is affected by the total personality and experience of the employee receiving the message, feedback is important. Simply stated, you don't really know what you have communicated until you have received feedback. Feedback should be considered a way of giving help. It is essential information supplied by others to help a person discover his effectiveness as a communicator. Feedback can be either corrective or confirming—an employee needs both. With a continual flow of reliable feedback, the supervisor can determine whether he or she is "on target" and can make any necessary changes.

Feedback can tell the receiver how his or her behavior appears to others or affects the feelings of others. The individual is free to use or not use the feedback.

Feedback is not evaluative. It is focused on specific behavior, not on the quality of the person. By avoiding personal evaluation, there is no need for the individual to act defensively. Everyone's perception of other people is somewhat distorted. Therefore, feedback from one person should always be checked against feedback from others.

A little feedback is better than none at all, but the more feedback the better. The supervisor should not limit the employee to simple yes or no responses, but rather encourage open responses and questions.

LISTENING: THE LOST ART

If there is one area where the modern supervisor fails, it is in communication. Communication is the best way to reach agreement on an institution's objectives and direct efforts toward meeting those objectives. A point made in Chapter Two bears repeating here. In an American Management Association study of superior-subordinate communication at the managerial level,[5] researchers found:

> If a *single* answer can be drawn from this detailed study into superior-subordinate communication on the managerial level ..., it is this: If one is speaking of the subordinate's specific job—his duties, the requirements he must fulfill in order to do his work well, his intelligent anticipation of future changes in his work, and the obstacles which prevent him from doing as good a job as possible—he and his boss do not agree, in almost every area...

Over the years I have become convinced that we waste energy and economic resources concentrating on the *form* of communication rather than the *substance*. For years I engaged in the counterproductive habit of seeking driving directions at gas stations or from a pedestrian or another driver, and rode away without having absorbed the instructions. *I had not listened.* Half the process of communication is listening—not just sitting *back* and listening, but sitting *up* and listening. The old cliché "what we have here is a failure to communicate" can be paraphrased, "what we have here is the result of poor listening habits."

The better listener a supervisor is, the better listening he or she will inspire. Here are some tips on improving listening habits that will work for you and for your coworkers:

1. Most of us talk too much. We spend too much time explaining our own position at the expense of understanding where the other person stands. Use judicious silence. At the beginning of a discussion, confine

yourself to asking questions. Remain silent for a period of time after each question is posed. Silence is a great way to motivate the other person to speak up. The best way to gauge your own listening capacity is to time your periods of silence.

2. Most of us frame questions to get the answers we *want* to hear, so try this—use open-ended questions. Frame your questions so that you leave the way open for whatever type of answer the other person truly wants to give. Allow the person to finish the answer. At the point you initially think the speaker is finished, just grunt or nod a little and let the speaker continue, just in case he or she has something additional to say.

3. Most of us set up communication in a counterproductive atmosphere. Schedule discussions of problems when the facts and details are fresh in everyone's mind. Pick a time and a place that provides minimum distraction and maximum comfort. If the situation is emotion-laden, provide for a cooling-off period. Most important, protect the dignity of all parties to the communication process.

4. Much communication is done on an ad hoc basis with little advance preparation. Save yourself a lot of time and aggravation by checking records and investigating facts ahead of time. It might be helpful to request a detailed report from your subordinate in advance of a meeting. The report can serve as a point of departure for the discussion.

5. Many of us let emotional filters get in the way of understanding. Be honest about your biases. When you feel strongly about a subject, be particularly careful. At such times there is more chance for you to misinterpret, misunderstand, and miscommunicate. One way you can guard against "emotional" listening is to have another listener present, a resource person. The next time your emotions boil over, make a mental note regarding the time and place and people involved. You might be able to track down the source of your feelings and the trigger that sets you off.

6. Most of us listen only for facts. We fail to see the subject from the other person's point of view. Listen for *feelings*. Pay as much attention to the way you or someone else says things as to what is said. A good way to perfect your listening for feelings is to deliberately put aside the facts and details of the presentation, dig deeply, and listen to the *overall* approach. Then check out your impressions with these phrases: "I conclude that you approve (or disapprove) of ..." or "Am I right in concluding that what you are saying is ..."

Communication is the prime tool of the modern supervisor and probably the most difficult one to perfect. The communications process is complicated because there are so many different messages involved. It has been suggested that each communication involves at least six messages:

1. What you *mean* to say.
2. What you *actually* say.
3. What the other person *hears*.
4. What the other person *thinks* he hears.
5. What the other person *says*.
6. What you *think* the other person says.

How do you attempt to deal with this? Here's a suggestion to use the next time you are in a discussion, a debate, or an argument. Before you reply to the other person's comments, *repeat* what the other person said. Before the other person replies to your comment, he or she should repeat what you have said. It will be both an eye- and ear-opener!

GAINING COOPERATION IS HALF THE BATTLE

More often than not, change requires cooperation. There are few instances where a single individual can develop and implement a specific change. The need for cooperation is underscored. If there is an area of supervisory skill which should be honed to perfection, it is the supervisor's responsibility to gain cooperation to ensure a smooth and expeditious transition from the old to the new.

One expert suggests the following skills which, when applied, can create a spirit of effective teamwork.

1. *Avoid arguments.* Understand what the other person is concerned about and listen beyond the emotions. This, of course, requires letting the other person tell the full story without interruption. Criticism should be minimized. Criticizing your subordinate may win you the battle, but you will certainly lose the war. The key to gaining agreement is to move from small points of consensus to overall and final agreement on the totality of the change.

2. *Admit your errors.* We are all vulnerable and very few of us can state that we are never wrong. It is well to remember that people do not like others who are "always right." Admitting your mistakes when they are made will gain you immeasurable respect from your subordinates.

3. *Establish a receptive frame of mind.* This can be accomplished by explaining why the change has to be implemented and how it will benefit

all—yourself and your subordinates. Emphasize the need for cooperation and the essential role the subordinate plays in implementing the
change. Ask for ideas and suggestions on moving from present methods
to new methods. Receptivity seldom comes by fiat—you cannot legis-
late a receptive frame of mind. The supervisor's task is to develop conditions that will encourage the subordinate to listen and be objective.
Once you have established this receptive frame of mind you can rest
assured your subordinates will be cooperative.

4. *A sympathetic "no" is better than a harsh "yes."* Gaining agreement
at any price is poor supervisory practice. You will have to say "no" at
times. More often than not, if "no" is said in a sympathetic and understanding way, it will not produce negative reactions. Use a friendly,
nonthreatening approach, show a sincere interest in the reactions of
your employees, explain the reasons for your "no," and finally, express
your appreciation.

5. *Dramatize ideas or suggestions.* Of all the senses, the sense of sight is
the strongest. Therefore, it is most helpful to dramatize the ideas or
suggestions for change by use of visual aids—including diagrams,
charts, and films.

6. *Set a fair challenge.* Your employees will normally rise to
challenges. A great deal of research has indicated that employees perform better and are more cooperative when they are presented with a
challenging goal.

7. *Praise in advance.* The need for appreciation stands at the top of the
pyramid of employee "wants." In the very complicated and hierarchical structures of most health care facilities, employees at the bottom
rung often feel like "invisible people." Praise should not be bestowed
grudgingly. Given the highly important work in health care facilities
and the day-to-day pressures, praise is vital. Supervisors will reply,
"There just isn't enough time," but the successful supervisor is able to
find something to commend in even the least competent person.

8. *Don't demand cooperation.* It just is not possible to force people to
cooperate. At most, you will get surface cooperation. True cooperation
can come only on a voluntary basis.[6]

WORKER PARTICIPATION IN MANAGEMENT:
RESEARCH STUDIES

There is more and more evidence that when workers are allowed to
make some decisions about their own work, they will be more productive.
Most of the plans to increase worker participation attempt to develop a

spirit of cooperation and teamwork on the job. The same principle can be applied to the facilitating of change. Where subordinates are allowed to express themselves and decision making is shared between the supervisor and the subordinate— decision making more by consensus than by fiat— there is a marked reduction in rivalry and conflict and a greater sense of psychological success. Decisions reached by consensus have enormous positive effects on productivity. When subordinates have a voice in significant problem-solving activities and therefore more responsibility for their own and fellow-workers' futures, they often experience a greater sense of interdependence with themselves and the whole, an enlarged awareness of the whole, better time perspective, and greater capacity to change the organization's internal makeup. The same researcher cautions that unless the participants truly believe and behave in ways consistent with these new values, the "changes suggested ... will fail because they will be perceived by the subordinates for what they really are: gimmicks and techniques to manipulate people and ... place power in the hands of people who do not tend to trust one another or probably themselves."[7]

Research was done concerning the features of the hospital management structure that lead to alienation of nonsupervisory personnel, particularly testing the hypothesis that the degree of alienation is related to the degree to which nonsupervisory nursing personnel are allowed to participate in a management decision. The results indicated that alienation is greater in situations where nonsupervisory staff are not allowed to participate in the decision-making process, and that inflexible bureaucratic systems tend to cause frustrations and depersonalization of staff relations causing loss of initiative.[8]

The supervisor should encourage subordinates' participation in establishing criteria for group and individual performance. In this way, subordinates help determine the basis on which their efforts will be judged. Just as important, it involves subordinates in the planning process, which will increase their commitment to the agreed-upon goals and objectives.

Coch and French conducted a study in a factory. The study dealt with overcoming resistance to change. There were three groups: Group 1 was the control group. Group 2 featured participation by representatives of the workers in designing job changes. Group 3 featured total participation by all members of the group.

In the case of Group 1, the control group, the production department modified the job, set the new piece rate, and then held a group meeting to communicate the change. Workers were told that the change was necessary because of competitive conditions, and the new piece rate was explained by the time-study man. Questions were answered. The results were disappointing: the group restricted production. This was related to the group's overall rejection of a change they saw as arbitrary and unreasonable.

In Group 2, the plant manager met with representatives of the group and there was joint planning. Again the competitive picture was pursued. The representatives were exposed to a dramatic presentation of the change. Two identical garments were displayed. The group was asked to identify the cheaper one and they could not. Yet one of the garments was produced the year before and the other was new. It was clearly explained and dramatically presented that the new garment was the cheaper one. The management presented its plan for change and the new piece rate. The representatives were informed of the need to eliminate all unnecessary work. Several operators were trained in the new methods and a piece rate agreeable to the representatives of the group was set. The results? Within two weeks productivity was satisfactory and met the competitive needs.

In Group 3, the plant manager met with individual workers. *Every worker was involved in meetings and every worker was consulted.* The methods used in Group 2 were also used, but here every worker participated. In a matter of days this group reached peak efficiency. The findings suggest that broad participation and planning for change reduce resistance dramatically.[9]

THE TALKING CHIEFS

Merrihue starts his book on communications with an apocryphal story:

Ganduki was a newly chosen warrior chieftain of an African tribe in a remote fastness in the vast Belgian Congo. Much irked by the poaching and sporadic raids of a persistent chief in a rival tribe, Ganduki called together his warriors and after a six day march, liquidated the troublesome tribe in a brilliant coup distinguished by its strategy and his personal courage. On the long trek home, Ganduki was sorely troubled despite the great victory and the booty and the slaves his warriors were bringing back. A man of action, but inarticulate, he would rather wage another battle than face up to the victory speech his tribe would expect upon his return. So calling upon his medicine man, Bo-Gobi, he prevailed upon him to communicate the magnitude and the brilliance of the victory to the homefolks.

And so it was. After hours of feasting, Bo-Gobi mounted an ivory dais and began the narrative of the battle. As he warmed to his task to the rising crescendo of the throbbing drums, the gaudily painted, spear-waving warriors leaped and howled in the eerie light cast by the roaring fire and when he had completed his tale, Bo-Gobi was caught up in the arms of his tribesmen and with a mighty shout, they hailed him as their savior and newly elected chief.[10]

Clear enough? The chiefs who master the ability to talk—to communicate—are accepted as true leaders. Your skill as a communicator is essential to your success as a supervisor and to the productivity of your work crew. No matter how varied your activities may be and how specialized your skills are, in the final analysis the success of every supervisor is related to communication. Essentially the supervisor gets work done through other people, and to accomplish this the supervisor must communicate effectively.

You must be especially careful about upward communication. Your subordinates often tell you what they think you want to hear. They will minimize incidents that will result in your "vindictiveness" or "unhappiness." If you want to obtain accurate information, you must develop an organizational style based on trust and confidence—one that invites a free flow and exchange of information up and down the line. Don't assume that subordinates share your contentment and satisfaction with the organization. Too often people tend to hear what they want to hear and close their ears to what they do not want to hear. If you are to obtain honest and objective communication from your subordinates, they have got to believe that you are operating with honesty and objectivity. Has what you've told them in the past been accurate, open, and factual? Can they rely on your word?

You never communicate in a vacuum. Effective communication flows from sound employee relations. If your subordinates believe that you do not play favorites, that you do not take all the credit, that you do not pass the buck, that you do back them up, that you are fair and dependable, they will listen to what you have to say.

HOW TO PRODUCE MORE EFFECTIVE COMMUNICATION

Merrihue suggests that if you as a first-line supervisor hope to meet the universal standards for effective communications with your employees, you will first need to:

1. Gain the confidence of your employees by:

    a. being impartial and consistent,

    b. making no commitments that you cannot fulfill,

    c. making certain that all problems and grievances are answered promptly and correctly,

    d. making the employees' work problems your own—and actively representing your employees' interest to other levels of management,

    e. making it clear that the institution has grievance machinery that works!

2. Gain the respect and the friendship of your employees by:

    a. according respectful treatment to each employee as an individual and esteemed associate, showing sincere interest in their welfare,

    b. displaying enthusiasm over their progress,

    c. being considerate and helpful in all possible ways,

    d. demonstrating your sincere personal interest in matters that are important to them—attending weddings, funerals, delivering pay and benefit checks in person when they are ill, attending social affairs together, family nights, etc.

3. Having thus established the proper climate for good downward communication to receptive employees and good upward communication from employees who feel free to discuss matters with you, you will need to develop your skills in:

    a. listening,

    b. talking,

    c. selling.

4. Of all the skills you will need to develop, none is more important than the ability to listen carefully in order to achieve full understanding of the information received, to take action quickly based on this understanding, and to communicate the results of such action to the individuals involved.[11]

I suggest that you ask yourself these six questions before you attempt to communicate to your employees:

1. Do I assume that if an idea is clear to me it will be clear to the receiver? (Just not so!)

2. Do I make it comfortable for others to tell me what is really on their minds—or do I encourage them to tell me only what I would like to hear? (It had better be the former!)

3. Do I check my understanding of what another person has told me before I reply? (Feedback is essential to effective communication!)

4. Am I tolerant of other people's feelings, realizing that their feelings, which may be different from mine, affect their communication? (We are always dealing with human emotions!)

5. Do I really try to listen from the sender's point of view before evaluating the message from my point of view? (There are two people in most conversations; the other person has a point of view!)

6. Do I make a conscious effort to build a feedback mechanism into all communications since even at its best, communication is an imperfect process? (Did he or she hear what I meant to say?)

With the advent of large institutions and complex delivery systems, the modern supervisor is equipped with techniques and methods far superior to his predecessor . . . but we all have paid a high price for this specialization. In an era of "over-specialization," we no longer do the jobs ourselves; we as supervisors differ from our earlier counterpart, and from the present workers inasmuch as we must get the job done through others. To the extent that we develop and refine the art of communication, we will be effective supervisors.

PRINCIPLES OF EFFECTIVE COMMUNICATION

We communicate in many ways: orally—in face-to-face-communications with our employees; by memorandum; by bulletins—on bulletin boards; at meetings—in conference form, in lecture form, with or without group participation. There is no question that successful organizations are successful in the area of communications. No matter what form communication takes, there is a sender and there is a receiver. The sender needs a receiver who will tune into the message and/or who can clear up the static. These are some underlying principles for effective employee-supervisor communication:

1. Communication should not be regarded as a tool or "helping" aspect of the organization, but as the essence of organized activity and the basic process from which all other functions derive.

2. Communication should be subject to the same controls as other organizational activities—that is, the accepted management principles of analysis planning, coordination, evaluation.

3. Communication should be thought of as directional—upward, downward, or horizontal from the sender.

4. Ineffective communication can mean wasted time and resources and, therefore, can result in lower productivity and higher costs.

5. We communicate in a variety of ways, verbal and nonverbal (through gestures, facial expressions, body postures and movements, tone of voice, and dress). Most of all we communicate by our actions.

6. People will generally hear, read, observe, and choose to understand only those parts of a message that relate to their own interests, desires, and needs.

7. One cannot *not* communicate. When a response is expected and is not forthcoming, silence communicates fear, stubbornness, uncooperativeness, and so on. Thus, our choice is not between communicating or not communicating, but between communicating effectively and ineffectively, between contributing or not contributing to organizational goals.

8. Although many supervisors feel that a message need be transmitted only once, specialists insist that repetition is important.

9. Communication is generally more effective when it provides the means for "feedback." Without feedback the sender cannot know what effect the message has had on the receiver's behavior, nor can the sender know how to achieve better communication next time. Communications which provide for feedback are called "two-way communications."

10. Although effective communication requires an expert use of media, the greatest barrier to communication probably lies in the area of human relations. Communication does not occur merely because *a message is sent;* it must also *be received* with reasonable fidelity.[12]

Key Points on How to Communicate the Change

1. As a supervisor you must initiate changes at a faster rate than ever before.

2. Most employees react to change with resistance. Understand that resistance and work with it.

3. To minimize resistance, explain in advance the need for change, gain consensus, and establish a receptive frame of mind.

4. Don't personalize the change. Indicate clearly and dramatically how the change will benefit the individual and the group.

5. Effect a feedback loop. Make sure that you are "on target." Remember that what you *mean* to say is not always what you *actually* say or what the other person *hears*. Feedback is a method of establishing

understanding. It is a mirror, not a directive. Feedback is possible only when the subordinate believes he or she can be frank and honest.

6. Half the process of communication is listening. The better listener a supervisor is, the better listening he or she will inspire.

7. People who participate in the shaping of change are more likely to be receptive to the change and, therefore, more productive. Increased participation in decision making can be an effective management tool, depending on the management style which has preceded it. If your subordinates believe that you truly value their ideas, that you will consider their suggestions objectively, that they can be free to voice their concerns to you—then and only then will participation be effective.

NOTES

1. Willard V. Merrihue, *Managing by Communication* (New York: McGraw-Hill Company, 1960), p. 243.

2. Leo B. Moore, "Too Much Management, Too Little Change," *Harvard Business Review,* January-February 1956, p. 41.

3. W. G. Bennis, K. D. Benne, and R. Chin, *The Planning of Change* (New York: Holt, Rinehart and Winston, 1964), passim.

4. P. Ecker, et al., *Handbook for Supervisors* (Englewood Cliffs, N.J.: Prentice-Hall, Inc., 1959), pp. 167-169.

5. N. R. S. Maier, et al., *Superior-Subordinate Communication in Management, Research Study No. 52* (New York: American Management Association, 1961), p. 9.

6. Alfred R. Lateiner, *Modern Techniques of Supervision* (Stamford, Conn.: Lateiner Publishing), originally appearing in *The Technique of Supervision* by Alfred R. Lateiner (New London, Conn.: National Foremen's Institute, 1954), pp. 28-29.

7. Chris Agyris, *The Integration of the Individual in the Organization—Social Science Approaches to Business Behavior* (Homewood, Ill.: Dorsey Press, 1962), pp. 85-87.

8. Jeanne Laporte, *Participatory Management—The Technique to Alleviate Alienation of Bureaucratic Organizations,* Thesis: University of Ottawa, Ontario, May 1972.

9. L. Coch and J. R. P. French, "Overcoming Resistance to Change" in Down Cartwright and Alvin Zander, eds., *Group Dynamics: Research and Theory,* 2nd ed. (Evanston, Ill.: Row Peterson and Company, 1960), passim.

10. Merrihue, *op. cit.,* p. 1.

11. *Ibid.,* pp. 108-109

12. *Improving Employee-Management Communication in Hospitals, A Special Study in Management Practices and Problems* (New York: Training Research and Special Studies Division, United Hospital Fund, 1965).

Chapter 6

How To Discipline:
The Positive Approach

If you are a supervisor you are going to be faced, almost daily, with the need to effect corrective action when an employee is chronically late, has an absentee problem, disregards a rule or policy of the institution, refuses to follow an order, is unproductive, is uncooperative, or in some way does not meet the standards of the institution. Taking corrective action is often a euphemism for discipline. On the other hand, the goal of positive discipline is to salvage the employee, to correct the behavioral pattern that is either antisocial or anti-institution.

More often than not, the act of disciplining is conceived of as punishment. Such an approach is referred to as negative discipline. Punishment may be the least effective way to discipline. We shall deal here with the complete spectrum of *constructive* discipline.

A CASE STUDY IN EFFECTIVE DISCIPLINARY ACTION

"You just can't fire anyone here. The union won't permit it." A physician at a large medical center voiced this complaint to the personnel director. The physician referred to "the good old days" when the hospital was run by the doctors and administrators. Now she felt it was run by the union.

The physician was talking specifically about an employee in her department who she felt was beyond redemption. Since she had concluded that she could not terminate him, she offered a proposal to the personnel director that in effect would "neutralize" the unsatisfactory employee. Instead of releasing him, she was going to keep him in drydock.

Earlier that day a hearing had been held in the personnel director's office in which the union appealed the termination of one of its members, who also happened to be a union delegate. The hearing lasted almost two hours. At the conclusion, the termination was upheld—the union concurred in this decision. But didn't that physician say that you couldn't fire anyone? Wherein lies the difference?

In the first case, a look at the employee's folder revealed no warning notices, no negative performance evaluations, no record of unsatisfactory performance. The physician who headed the department asserted loudly and clearly that the employee was inefficient, often late, often absent, surly, and insubordinate. Yet not a line of documentation existed to support these accusations!

In the case of the union delegate who had been with the institution for three years, the personnel folder contained several warning notices, a notice of suspension, and a final warning notice. In addition, the performance evaluation reflected specific problems—clearly enumerated with dates—regarding attendance, punctuality, and attitude.

The supervisor who said "You can't fire anyone here..." was pronouncing a self-fulfilling prophecy. Believing this notion, she documented nothing. She was guilty of the cardinal sin in employee discipline—offering innocuous performance evaluations to escape the unpleasantness of that "chore." Many hospital supervisors will not admit their unwillingness to take the time or effort to discipline, to face the unpleasant job of counseling, issuing warning notices, and confronting the employee in a hearing which could result in a suspension or discharge.

The truth of the matter is that the doctor was right. She was not able to fire anyone for a capricious or arbitrary reason, or where just cause could not be established. For other than clearly overt acts of insubordination, refusal to follow a direct order, or acts which endanger or compromise good patient care, the supervisor has the responsibility of documenting his or her case. *This in no way means that the supervisor is unable to act.* It simply means he or she must show that the employee was fully cognizant of the problems and that a pattern of warnings was used to denote progressive disciplining.

GOOD AND JUST CAUSE

The burden of providing "good and just cause" for discipline rests on administration. If cause has been proved, a penalty imposed by the administration will not be modified by an arbitrator, unless it is shown to have been clearly arbitrary, capricious, discriminatory, or excessive in relation to the offense. The key point to understand about limitation on the right to discipline is that administration may discipline up through discharge *only* for sufficient and appropriate reasons.

It behooves the administration to develop a sound procedure, based upon due process, for the discipline of unionized employees. Even if it is not mandated by a collective bargaining agreement, due process should be available to all employees. Arbitrators will normally support a management action if progressive discipline includes, first, a verbal reprimand and full explanation of what is necessary to remedy the situation, followed by written reprimand for a second infraction and a clear warning of the future penalties that may be imposed. A final warning and suspension may follow, and subsequently the ultimate penalty of discharge.

The arbitrator will also consider whether or not the employee was fully aware of the standards against which his or her behavior was measured. These standards include basic rules and regulations that outline offenses which subject employees to disciplinary action, and the extent of such disciplinary action.

Disciplining has become more juristic and legalistic with the advent of a union, but that does not mean that it is impossible to discipline employees. It does mean that the administration must record actual events, offenses, and transgressions. You cannot simply wish away problem employees.

Jules Justin, a prominent labor arbitrator, lists some noteworthy rules of corrective discipline:

1. Discipline to be meaningful must be corrective, not punitive.

2. When you discipline one, you discipline all.

3. Corrective discipline satisfies the rule of equality of treatment by enforcing equally among all employees established rules, safety practices, and responsibility on the job.

4. It is the job of the supervisor, not the shop steward, to make the worker toe the line or increase efficiency.

5. Just cause or any other comparable standard for justifying disciplinary action under the labor contract consists of three parts:

a. Did the employee breach the rule or commit the offense charged against him?

b. Did the employee's act or misconduct warrant corrective action or punishment?

c. Is the penalty just and appropriate to the act or offense as corrective punishment?

6. **The** burden of proof rests on the supervisor. He or she must justify each of the three parts that make up the standard of just cause under the labor contract.[1]

FORMS OF DISCIPLINE

The real purpose of discipline is to correct employees so that unacceptable behavior does not recur. In addition, you wish to deter others from committing the same errors. We have learned a great deal about the need for progressive disciplinary action. Most of what we have learned has come from two sources—the behavioral scientists and arbitrators.

Arbitrators tell us what is required to sustain a discharge. The following points were enunciated by a prominent arbitrator, Milton Friedman, but many other arbitrators have set up similar criteria for the sustaining of discharges.

1. The employer must prove that the alleged acts occurred and were of sufficient gravity to warrant termination.
2. The employer must show that the misconduct was not condoned, but the employee was specifically warned of the consequences through progressive discipline, such as written warnings and suspension.
3. The evidence must demonstrate that the employee made no genuine effort to heed the warnings although the consequences of continued misconduct were known.
4. The employee cannot be singled out for disparate treatment for offenses that do not subject others to similar discipline.
5. When a long-service employee is involved, there must be sound cause to believe that the events are not transitory, but form a consistent and recurrent pattern that is unlikely to change in the future.

The Oral Reprimand

It is clear that progressive disciplining usually starts with oral reprimands or oral warnings. This function is often handled in a counseling session. What is the purpose of the action? It should be to nip in the bud behavior that is inappropriate to the work area. The necessary ingredients for a successful counseling encounter are complete privacy, a well planned agenda, enough time to arrive at agreement, and a positive attitude on the part of the supervisor.

In such sessions employees should receive a complete outline of the action in question. Details should not be spared, and dates and times and places should be communicated. The specific institution policy or rule in question should be enunciated. The specific documents (such as a union contract or the personnel policy manual) wherein such rules are contained should be examined. The employee should be given complete freedom to answer the charge, explain his or her behavior, admit or deny the action.

It is obvious that an effective counseling session will develop from the point that the employee *agrees that the action occurred and was inappropriate.* If such an agreement is reached, a plan to improve the employee's performance should be discussed. As I mentioned in an earlier chapter, it is also important at this time to acknowledge the positive aspects of the employee's behavior.

After the counseling session has been completed, anecdotal notes should be prepared by the supervisor and placed in the employee's folder *in the department.* It is not appropriate at this point to forward such notes to the personnel department for inclusion in the employee's personnel folder.

We must repeat that the supervisor who wishes to effect corrective disciplining should be more interested in changing an employee's behavioral patterns and attitudes than in reprimanding that employee. Lateiner[2] offers some pointers to the supervisor interested in making criticism more constructive:

1. Don't reprimand a worker who is angry or excited. Wait until he or she has cooled down. Wait until you cool down, too.

2. Don't bawl out someone in front of other people. This is embarrassing and humiliating and is likely to do more harm than good.

3. Find out how the worker feels and thinks about the situation. If you want someone to do something differently, you first have to find out what she or he already knows.

4. When you criticize a person, it is much better to compare her or his performance to department standards than to the performance of another employee. A person is more likely to feel resentful or insecure if she or he is compared unfavorably to a coworker.

5. Most important, if you reprimand constructively, you must show a person how to improve his or her performance. You don't want to destroy an employee's self-confidence. You want to build up confidence by guiding the worker in the direction of a satisfactory performance.

The oral reprimand or warning interview is a useful way for the supervisor to establish a sound relationship with *all* employees—those who require such warnings and those who do not. Employees normally respect supervisors who apply the rules of the institution fairly. Although criticism is often a disturbing element, the need for *constructive* criticism can be fully appreciated by employees.

If the supervisor is to discipline firmly and wisely, it is essential that the employee relations administrator or personnel director fully support the supervisor in those instances where institutional policy is being protected and carried out. It is equally important that the department head or director of the institution provide clear evidence that the supervisor will be backed up at crucial moments. This does not mean that there will never be a situation where the supervisor is overruled, but such incidences should not be based on political pressures, legal technicalities, or sentimentality. The responsibility of meting out discipline is difficult enough without undercutting the first-line supervisor.

Before concluding our discussion of the oral reprimand or warning interview, it should be made clear that the oral reprimand is not appropriate or effective in the face of flagrant offenses such as insubordination, theft, fighting, or carrying firearms. Such actions call for sharper responses—often termination.

Warning Notices

Overt flaunting of institutional rules and appropriate behavior patterns is dealt with by the first-line supervisor either by means of a formal warning notice, suspension, or discharge—if, and only after, a formal warning interview has been held. (This proscription does not apply if the transgression is a major and flagrant one such as those mentioned under exceptions to the oral reprimand.) Some examples of negative behavior which may call for a written warning notice are:

- Insubordination or impertinence
- Unauthorized or chronic absenteeism
- Chronic lateness
- Loafing or sleeping
- Misrepresentation of time cards or records
- Drinking alcoholic beverages
- Dishonesty
- Fighting on the job
- Gambling

The warning notice should not come as a surprise to an employee. It is essentially the second step in the arsenal of weapons used to reverse a poor behavioral pattern. It is often preceded by the oral reprimand, but may directly follow a clear violation of institutional rules and regulations. In preparing the warning notice, the supervisor is again concerned with facts and not with subjective opinions.

The institution normally provides a form to be used for written warning notices. This form usually calls for a clear statement of the specific rule or policy that has been violated. The supervisor may have to refer to the union contract or personnel policy manual or written bulletin containing the specific rule.

Following this reference point, the written warning notice should move toward a description of the act in question. Once again the supervisor is urged to be specific and complete. Dates, time, and, where appropriate, witnesses should be included.

Now we come to the most important part of the warning notice—a statement to indicate that immediate satisfactory improvement must be shown and maintained unless further disciplinary action is to be taken. In many cases, this "immediate satisfactory improvement" can be outlined in detail. For example, suppose an employee has shown a pattern of absenteeism—let us say three days each month for the last six months (many of the days were Mondays, making three-day weekends possible). The supervisor will indicate that the employee's pattern of Monday absences is not acceptable, that the employee's attendance will be monitored over the next two, three, or four months to gauge improvement, and that if there is no improvement, the employee will be subject to suspension and possible termination.

The warning notice is presented to the employee in private. If possible, the employee should be asked to sign the warning notice, acknowledging receipt. More important than this acknowledgment of the warning form is the employee's acknowledgment that the behavior is inappropriate and that improvement is forthcoming. In some cases—more often than not where unions are involved—employees will refuse to sign a warning notice form. This should be expected and understood, but the supervisor's responsibility does not end here. The supervisor, in order to emphasize the importance of the action and ensure the "legality" of the presentation, should ask another supervisor to witness the actual reading and offer a copy of the warning notice to the employee. This is necessary only if the employee refuses to sign the warning notice form.

Despite the discussion above, it is important to remember that the supervisor's cardinal responsibility in this procedure is to attempt a restructuring of the employee's behavior; it is not the primary responsibility or objective to punish the employee.

One bit of advice is necessary before we explore the final two steps in the disciplinary arsenal of weapons—suspension and termination. There is no easy panacea that can be offered in the area of behavior control. In a few cases oral reprimands or warning notices will never be enough. In still more cases suspensions may be counterproductive. The supervisor must keep in mind that constructive disciplining is a means of achieving the end product—a change in behavior patterns.

Suspension

The suspension is not universally accepted as an effective way to correct behavior patterns. Many employees find the suspension a respite from the stress of the work area. *Some employees even enjoy being out on strike.* For an employee with a chronic absentee record a suspension is certainly not the worst sort of punishment.

A one-day suspension can be as effective as a one-week suspension. The shock of the suspension will usually bring the employee to his or her senses. The length of the suspension has little effect on the probability of rehabilitation. Very often the suspension of an employee causes inordinate difficulties in scheduling and in meeting production quotas. I have come to the conclusion that a one- or two-day suspension is a sufficient final warning to employees before termination. The suspension should be accompanied with a written warning notice indicating prior attempts, both informal and formal, toward rehabilitation. Most important, the suspension should indicate that it constitutes the final warning.

Termination

In order to sustain a discharge where an arbitration procedure is available, the following minimal requirements must be met. In fact, these requirements should be operative whether or not there is an arbitration procedure, whether or not there is a union.

1. Facts must be presented, clearly indicating that the employee actually committed the offense. Opinion must be separated from hard documentation. Witnesses may be essential.
2. You must be able to display a consistent approach to the offense in question: no playing of favorites.
3. The record should indicate a progressive disciplining ladder, except in the case of blatant and serious offenses.
4. The punishment must fit the crime.

Progressive disciplining normally must precede the discharge of an employee. The procedure for progressive disciplining as outlined above includes a verbal reprimand and a full explanation of what is necessary to remedy the situation. Normally a second infraction calls for a written reprimand with a clear warning of future penalties which may be imposed. A suspension may follow with a final warning and the ultimate penalty is discharge. There is a further consideration in cases that involve discharge—*consistency.* A double standard is often found in health care institutions: one standard for the medical staff and another standard for the other employees. We shall not explore this provocative subject, but the supervisor should be aware of the possibility of employee complaints to the union and to outside agencies of disparate treatment of professionals and nonprofessionals.

DISCIPLINING FOR OPTIMUM RESULTS

Much of the debate over appropriate discipline concerns the spirit, extent, or degree of enforcement that brings optimum results. Pfiffner and Fels put this critical question in proper focus:

> Should discipline be strict and severe or tolerant and easygoing? The answer will not be found by locating the optimum point between strict and easy, but rather in the fundamental nature of the social organization which the supervisor must understand as part of his disciplining duties. If the basic mores of an organization are developed in a manner that commands the respect and conformance of its members, disciplining should offer no special problem. The rank and file member will observe the mores either automatically or because of the pressures exerted to do so by other members of the group. That is, he probably will if he has a feeling of belonging and thus recognizing that to belong requires a contribution in accordance with his means and talents. Thus, in essence, the supervisor's attempts to discipline must see discipline as a means not of immediately stopping an undesirable behavior only, but of reaching a goal of desirable citizenship.[3]

Key Points to Effective Disciplining

1. Your primary concern in disciplining employees is to salvage them, *not* to scrap them.
2. Although punishment is part of disciplinary action, it is not the primary part.

3. Direct your attention, and therefore your plan of action, toward correcting improper employee actions.

4. Don't play favorites; be consistent; the rule of equality of treatment should pervade all your disciplinary actions.

5. In the final analysis, you (the supervisor) are responsible for maintaining appropriate employee behavioral patterns and productivity.

6. Whether or not the employees in your department are unionized, *just cause* must be established for all disciplinary action.

7. Be it ever so trite, the punishment must fit the crime.

8. Progressive disciplining includes oral reprimands (including counseling), written warnings, and suspensions; termination is defensible where the infraction or behavior was serious (theft, fighting, carrying firearms) or was preceded by the aforementioned steps.

9. Self-discipline develops where employees trust the supervisor and the management, where employees feel that their job is important and appreciated, where employees feel that they belong.

10. Positive discipline encompasses the following sound supervisory practices:[4]

a. Inform *all* employees of the rules and the penalties. The "why" of the rule is just as important as the "what."

b. Don't play the game of "Do as I say, not as I do." Set a good example. Employees look to their supervisors for fairness in application of the rules.

c. Don't jump before you look. Get all the facts. Keep uppermost in your mind the old adage that there are always *at least* two sides to every story.

d. Beware of incomplete facts or appearances. Judge the act within its context. Look for the least obvious motives and reasons.

e. Move quickly but not hastily. Don't let selected instances of misbehavior develop into habits.

f. Discipline—corrective, that is!—should be meted out in private.

g. Objectivity and fairness are *two* hallmarks of positive, corrective disciplinary action.

h. Consistency is the *third* hallmark.

i. Throughout the disciplinary process, keep your eye on the goal of the process: to correct improper behavior and to salvage the employee.

j. Use punishment as the last resort.

NOTES

1. Jules J. Justin, *How to Manage with a Union, Book One* (New York: Industrial Relations Workshop Seminars, Inc., 1969), pp. 294-295, 301-302.

2. Alfred R. Lateiner, *Modern Techniques of Supervision* (Stamford, Conn.: Lateiner Publishing), originally appearing in *The Technique of Supervision* by Alfred R. Lateiner, (New London, Conn.: National Foreman's Institute, 1954), pp. 28-39.

3. John M. Pfiffner and Marshall Fels, *The Supervision of Personnel,* 3rd ed. (Englewood Cliffs, N.J.: Prentice-Hall, Inc., 1964), pp. 111-112.

4. A special note of gratitude to Ms. Rita Hubert, graduate student in the Masters Program for Health Care Administration of Rensselaer Polytechnic Institute.

5. Developed by Dr. Leslie M. Slote.

Exhibit 2   Checklist for Corrective Action[5]

What is the past record of the employee?	Was the employee disciplined previously for the same type of offense? When? Should he or she receive a more severe penalty than a first offender?
Have you all the facts?	Refer to personnel records. Get concrete facts about this specific situation; refer to rules, standards, and policies; evaluate opinions and feelings. Was there an extenuating reason for the employee's behavior? (Sickness, money trouble, etc.)
Has the employee had a fair chance to improve? When?	Has he or she been given some help, advice, or explanation? Does he or she know what is expected? Did he or she know the rules and standards at the time of the infraction?
When was the employee first given a fair warning of the seriousness of his behavior?	Was a written record made and filed? Who gave the warning?

What action was taken in similar cases?

Are there others in your department who experienced different treatment under similar circumstances? In other departments?

What will be the effect of your action on the group?

Are you fully justified? What will be the effect on groups outside your department?

Are you going to handle this by yourself?

Should you clear with your boss or with the personnel director? Do you need assistance or further information? How is your timing?

What other possible actions are there?

Will your action help the hospital, help improve the work output in your department, and help the employee to improve? Should he or she be warned or suspended?

Chapter 7

How To Handle Grievances Effectively

The handling of employee grievances affords the supervisor the greatest opportunity to win over employee respect and gain employee confidence. The most important employer-employee relationship is the one that exists between the worker and his or her immediate supervisor. It is essential for supervisors to know their people, be genuinely interested in them, and recognize their needs and problems. This good relationship cannot only head off many grievances before they reach the formal grievance stage, but also lead to increased productivity.

The supervisor is often the day-to-day interpreter of institutional policy, rules, and regulations and the administrator of the union contract. If there is a Pandora's box in the day-to-day employer-employee relationship, it is the area of grievances. An unattended accumulation of minor irritations and aggravations may inflate and finally explode in the supervisor's face. A little bit of attention at the beginning will go further than a great deal of harried and pressured attention at the end. As a matter of fact, most complaints can be satisfactorily resolved by the supervisor before they become formal grievances.

A grievance may have some basis in fact or it may be fabricated or exaggerated beyond reality. A grievance may not truly be a grievance as defined in a union contract or under institutional policy. More often than not, it may be a gripe or just information-seeking on the part of the employee. In any case it must be dealt with and resolved.

MINIMIZING GRIEVANCES

Although there is no way to completely eliminate grievances, there are commonsense guidelines that will reduce the number and the cost of grievances. Here are some suggestions:

1. Be alert for common causes of irritation within your department. Correct minor irritations promptly before they explode into major problems.
2. Do not knowingly violate established policy, procedure, or practice. This, of course, requires the supervisor to be completely familiar with all policies and contractual clauses that affect the supervisor-employee relationship.
3. Keep promises. Do not make commitments you cannot keep. Many grievances are over the nonfulfillment of a commitment made by a supervisor.
4. Let your employees know how they are getting along. Don't wait for the formal performance review to keep an employee informed of progress or problems. This will minimize the number of grievances that develop when employees are warned about poor performance after having received positive performance reviews earlier in the year.
5. If an employee doesn't measure up, let that employee know. Find out why there is a problem and provide direction and coaching.
6. Encourage constructive suggestions; act on these suggestions where feasible and give proper recognition to the originators. Participation will go a long way to minimize grievances that may develop because of policy changes.
7. Assign and schedule work impartially; avoid favoritism in respect to working conditions or employee benefits.
8. Be sure your employees understand the meaning of and reasons for your orders and instructions. Use language that is meaningful from their point of view.
9. Be consistent in your words and actions unless there are important reasons for deviation. Where deviation is justified, clearly communicate those reasons to the employees. Explain changes in or deviations from policy, procedure, or established practice.
10. Act promptly on reasonable requests from your employees. Don't keep employees waiting for answers to their questions. Nothing is more destructive than a grievance allowed to grow because of lack of prompt response on the part of the supervisor. Remember, you may have to say "no," but a constructive and sympathetic "no" can do less damage than a harsh "yes."

11. If corrective action must be taken, take it promptly; but do not discipline an employee in public.

HEARING THE GRIEVANCE

Many gripes are not bona fide grievances because they concern situations not specifically covered by a union contract or by an institutional policy. Although a gripe may not qualify as a grievance, the employee should be heard on the subject. If a legalistic attitude is assumed at this stage and the gripes are dismissed summarily, hard feelings will be engendered and another issue properly subject to the grievance machinery will be used to exert pressure. It is not suggested that every petty gripe be given undue importance. However, the employee should not be brushed off without having the complaint fully heard.

Hearing a complaint requires attentive listening—get the complete facts and the underlying attitudes and feelings. Let the employee talk without interruption. Then ask questions until you are satisfied that you understand the specifics of the grievance and the true agenda. Do not become predisposed or argumentative in response to the employee's answers. Very often complaints reflect dissatisfaction in areas other than those under discussion. It is essential that you find out what is really bothering the employee—the hidden agenda. An excellent approach is to rephrase the employee's statement in your own words. This "reflection" serves four important purposes:

1. The employee is able to correct any misunderstanding you may have.
2. The employee has the opportunity to bring the complaint into closer focus.
3. You and the employee can assume that you understand the situation thoroughly.
4. The employee is assured that both of you are "on the same wave length," that you are empathetic and trying to understand the problem from the employee's point of view.

Further explanation or discussion should be reserved until after the facts have been checked, applicable policies and union contract provisions reviewed, and past practices, grievances, and commitments analyzed. Don't promise anything at this time other than a careful investigation. Specify a time within which an answer will be forthcoming. Don't mislead the employee by promising to do something about the complaint unless you are sure remedial action is in order.

There may be instances where a quick response is indicated. If you are absolutely certain of the facts, an immediate reply is in order. However, in most instances a hasty decision can be disastrous. If you are not sure of the facts, not sure of the appropriate policy provision or contract interpretation, or doubtful that the emotional climate is conducive to resolution, delay your response.

GETTING THE FACTS

After hearing and understanding the complaint, initiate an investigation. A complete investigation includes interviewing other employees who may have been involved, reviewing relevant records, and in general "stepping back" from the problem to gain objectivity. New facts and additional viewpoints are almost always uncovered in this way.

In your investigation, look for information concerning previous settlements of similar grievances and relevant policy or contract interpretations. You may call on other supervisors or the personnel manager. Precedent becomes very important. A hasty decision may provide a precedent with far-reaching impact. Many a supervisor has found that a hasty or careless decision over a relatively minor occurrence becomes important later in a different situation with more serious consequences. It is therefore essential that you investigate before you act.

DECISION-MAKING TIME

After analyzing all the facts uncovered by a thorough investigation, it is time to develop a solution to the problem and an answer to the grievance. It is a good idea to discuss your proposed solution with others. Checking out your hunch, your conclusion or your suggested options with others who are in a position to assess their probable impact is a wise idea. Ask your supervisor, the personnel manager, or other supervisors. Ask how this type of problem has been handled in the past. Consultation is a sign of caution, not indecision. You will not be criticized for reviewing your options with others if you have assembled the facts carefully and approached the grievance objectively.

Now it is time to put your answer in written form. Wherever possible, completely explain the reasons behind your decision. It is important that you deal with the specific complaint and not go beyond that complaint.

COMMUNICATING TO THE EMPLOYEE

Supervisors who admit to their mistakes are more respected than those who cover up mistakes. If a grievance has merit and an error has been made, admit this to the employee and indicate your intention to take immediate corrective action. Make certain that you take such corrective action.

If the complaint has no merit and the grievance is to be denied, a full explanation should be communicated to the employee. Attempt to gain the employee's understanding and acceptance of your decision. If the employee remains dissatisfied, don't get impatient and irritated. Appeals are normally provided for in institutional grievance procedures, and the procedure for such an appeal should be explained to the employee.

THE NEED FOR A WRITTEN RECORD

Whether a grievance is denied, granted, settled by compromise, or handled in another way, it is necessary to prepare a complete statement of all that occurred. Normally grievances are submitted on grievance forms which indicate the "disposition." Once completed the grievance form should be presented to the employee and a copy kept in the departmental files.

GENERAL GUIDELINES

The following points on effective grievance handling are important for the supervisor to review and accept:

1. There should be a strong desire to resolve dissatisfactions and conflicts before they become real problems.
2. Supervisors should empathize with their employees, try to understand employee problems, and be able and willing to listen in a nonjudgmental fashion.
3. The supervisor should have a sound working knowledge of personnel policy procedures and where appropriate, the union contract.
4. The supervisor must balance a personal commitment to the interests of the institution with a sense of fair play on behalf of the employees. The supervisor represents the employees to the administration and the administration to the employees.

Broadly speaking, the supervisor's responsibility in grievance procedures embraces four primary functions:

1. investigating the material facts,
2. analyzing the grievance to determine its basic causes,
3. discussing and answering the grievances, and
4. taking action to eliminate present problems and prevent future ones.

If you are to discharge your responsibilities properly, your first task upon receiving a grievance is to investigate, not evaluate.

Here are some of the ways to improve human relations when handling grievances:

1. *Be available.* Know your people are individuals and fit your methods to the individual. Cool off the hothead with patience; sense when something is troubling the quiet worker who keeps anger bottled up until it explodes; calm the sensitive employee who may think he or she is being slighted. You can't solve the problems of strangers, and unless you are approachable, you will have strangers working for you.

2. *Be relaxed.* When employees bring you gripes, real or fancied, let them sound off. If they see you are listening and will give them a fair hearing, the complaint won't look so big.

3. *Get the facts.* Get the story and get it straight. Ask questions to straighten out inconsistencies. Be objective and sympathetic.

4. *Investigate carefully.* Never accept hearsay. Find out for yourself the answers to such questions as who, what, when, where, and why. Check how the union contract or institutional policy covers the alleged offense, and review your files for precedence.

5. *Be tactful.* Many employees will start to tell a supervisor about unfair treatment only to realize halfway through their story that they don't have a real complaint. If supervisors help such employees "save face," the supervisor makes a friend. You never want a worker to leave the grievance interview humiliated and embarrassed.

6. *Act with deliberation.* Snap judgment leads to impulsive action. Take time to get all the facts. What caused the grievance? Where did it happen? Has the contract been violated? Has an institution policy been violated? Has the employee been unfairly treated? Has there been favoritism, unintentional or deliberate? Was this grievance related to others?

7. *Get the answer.* Maybe it is impossible to address the grievance immediately, but don't give employees the runaround. If you can't get the

facts you need to settle this case, say so. If the employee knows you are working on the problem, he or she is likely to be more reasonable.

8. *Consider the consequences of your decision.* Make sure you know the effect your settlement will have, not only on the individual, but on the group.

9. *Admit mistakes.* You are human and make mistakes, so if your decisions are occasionally reversed by higher ups, admit your error. Don't bear a grudge against the employee who was proved right at your expense.

10. *Sell your decisions.* When you deny an employee's grievance, explain why. A blunt "no" causes resentment. Don't pass the buck by blaming your denial on higher management. Supervision means leadership.[1]

LET'S LOOK AT SOME RESEARCH

First-line supervisors in ten unionized plants were studied by Jennings[2] to determine their attitudes toward the grievance procedure. He was looking at:

1. the significance of grievance handling as a supervisory responsibility,

2. the foremen's responsibilities and activities in grievance handling and

3. actions taken by other line- and staff-management officials in the grievance process.

He found the following:

1. Supervisors perceive that top management regarded grievance-handling responsibilities as an important aspect of the supervisor's job.

2. Supervisors did not consider the resolution of grievances extremely important.

3. When supervisors spent a great deal of effort resolving grievances, they did not feel they were given much credit for this activity.

4. A majority of the supervisors did not believe that they had the primary responsibility for the grievance procedure.

5. A majority believed that their grievance decisions were usually upheld by higher-level management.

6. A majority of foremen usually consulted the industrial relations representative before responding to a grievance.

What can we learn from the Jennings study? It appears that supervisors are not ranking grievance handling high enough in the total range of supervisory responsibilities. This may well have developed because upper management, although realizing the importance of that aspect of the supervisor's job, has not extended appreciation or recognition for that role. It seems essential that supervisors be given appropriate credit for minimizing and/or resolving grievances. Most arbitration cases (arbitration is usually the last step in a grievance procedure, wherein a third party not connected with the institution or the union judges the merits of the grievance and produces a binding decision) are won or lost on the basis of the supervisor's testimony. It is also obvious from the Jennings findings that communication with staff experts in industrial relations or employee relations is essential to producing consistent and defensible decisions.

A study by Turner and Robinson[3] examined the effect of grievance resolution on union-management relationships. Specifically, they examined the hypothesis that "the greater the number of grievances resolved at the lower steps of the grievance procedure, the more likely is a harmonious union-management relationship." Their findings supported the hypothesis.

To summarize, research indicates that upper management depends significantly on the first-line supervisor to resolve grievances. Yet supervisors seem not to give a high priority to this important responsibility. This would lead us to believe that supervisors do not fully realize that their role is fundamental in minimizing grievances and preventing a grievance from becoming a major dispute. Research data also indicate that the resolution of grievances in the lower steps of the grievance process leads to more harmonious labor-management relationships. The first-line supervisor is key to that improvement.

TIPS FOR HANDLING GRIEVANCES EFFECTIVELY

The principal requirements for handling grievances effectively are:

1. a strong desire to make the personnel policy manual and/or labor contract work, to resolve dissatisfactions and conflicts, and to supervise more effectively;
2. a strong effort on the part of first-line supervisors to settle grievances at the very first step in the grievance procedure;
3. a sound working knowledge of the personnel policy manual and the labor contract, including new interpretations and precedents;

4. a consistent approach to carrying out provisions of the personnel policy manual and/or labor contract.

You, the supervisor, play the key role in the handling of grievances. To be effective in that responsibility, heed the following advice:

1. The people who work for you are just that, people. Treat them as individuals.

2. It is essential that you maintain and preserve the dignity of the employee. This may be difficult when dealing with grievances, but it is at the heart of a sound supervisor-employee relationship.

3. Remember that employees want to be appreciated; they want to know that you recognize their meritorious performance. Give credit where it is due. This will minimize many grievances which spring from a lack of recognition.

4. Look to your employees for suggestions and advice. Give them the feeling that they are in on things. Many grievances arise because the employee is not prepared for change.

5. "A stitch in time. . . ." This old adage is most appropriate in effective grievance handling. Look around and try to anticipate areas and actions that may cause irritation. By anticipating problems you will minimize them.

6. Employees who are properly trained are less likely to have grievances. Employees who know what they are doing and, therefore, do it well, are less frustrated. This is of particular relevance when dealing with the new employee.

7. Unclear, unexplained orders or instructions can lead to grievances. Make certain that you communicate clearly and back up orders and instructions with a "why."

8. When you must administer discipline, be objective, equitable, and consistent. The majority of grievances stem from real or perceived inequality of treatment.

9. Don't belittle employees or underestimate them. If they have a grievance, it does not really matter whether it falls under the personnel policy manual or the labor contract. It is real to the employee and you must deal with it.

Key Points to Effective Handling of Grievances

1. Employees deserve a complete and empathetic hearing of all grievances they present.

2. The most important job in the handling of grievances is getting at the facts. Therefore, listen attentively, encourage a full discussion, and defer judgment.

3. Look for the hidden agenda. Look beyond the selected incident, judge the grievance in context.

4. Hasty decisions often backfire. On the other hand, the employee deserves a speedy reply. In order to determine the proper disposition of a grievance, ask yourself the following questions.
   a. What actually happened?
   b. Where did it happen?
   c. What should have happened?
   d. When did it happen?
   e. Who was involved?
   f. Were there any witnesses?
   g. Why did the problem develop?[4]

5. While you are investigating the grievance, try to separate fact from opinion or impressions. Consult others when appropriate. Most important, check with your personnel people.

6. After you have come to your decision, promptly communicate that decision to the employee. Remember, a sympathetic "no" is far more effective than a harsh "yes." Therefore, give the reason for the decision and inform the employee of the right to appeal.

7. Remember that you have to sell your decision. The decision is yours, don't pass the buck by placing the blame on your superiors.

8. There is no substitute for common sense in arriving at a decision.

9. Written records are most important, they serve as a review for the supervisor to ensure consistency.

10. Followup is essential. Even if the employee does not appeal your decision, you should check back to see if the decision "took" or was upheld. There is no better way to win employee respect than to give due recognition to employee problems. A little bit of followup goes a long way.

NOTES

1. This subsection was developed by Joseph Ferentino, Associate Director of Personnel, and Luther Thompson, Manager of Employee Relations, at The Mount Sinai Medical Center, New York City.

2. Ken Jennings, "Foremen's View of Their Involvement with Other Management Officials in the Grievance Process," *Labor Law Journal* 25, no. 25 (May 1974): 305-316.

3. James T. Turner and James W. Robinson, "A Pilot Study of the Validity of Grievance Settlement Rates as a Predictor of Union-Management Relations," *Journal of Industrial Relations,* 14, no. 3 (September 1972): 314-322.

4. J. Brad Chapman, "Constructive Grievance Handling," included in M. Gene Newport, ed., *Supervisory Management: Tools and Techniques* (New York: West Publishing Company, 1976), p. 268.

Chapter 8

How To Act or React To a Union Organizing Drive: What You Can Do

After almost three decades in the field of labor relations, I have come to the conclusion that what upper management does or doesn't do, what labor lawyers retained as consultants for institutions do or do not recommend, what the board of trustees believes should be the basic philosophy of the institution—all of these are not as significant as the effect of the first-line supervisor on employees' desire or lack of desire to take collective action. *More employees vote for or against their immediate supervisor than vote for or against the top administration, the board of trustees, or consultants.* It is at the day-to-day level of intercourse between the first-line supervisor and the employees that the institutional lifestyle impacts upon the rank-and-file employee; that impact is critical in a union organizing campaign. *Unions rarely organize employees; rather it is the administration's poor employee relations record (uppermost in that grouping is the first-line supervisor) that drives employees into unions.*

Management failure is the root cause of the majority of successful union campaigns. Management failure can include a lack of understanding of employee needs; a lack of competitiveness of salaries and fringe benefits; a lack of clear and usable communication lines; a lack of sound personnel policies; a lack of a formal and understandable grievance mechanism; a lack of appropriate and acceptable working conditions; the presence of arrogant, insensitive, overworked, and harried supervisors.

It is also patently clear that institutions that provide all the benefits and conditions of a union shop—with all the protection inherent in a union contract, such as seniority provisions, grievance and arbitration mechanisms, promotional opportunities—will not become unionized. It is the absence of these conditions plus the presence of insensitive management that *drives* employees into unions.

WHY PEOPLE JOIN UNIONS

There is a myth that outside rabble-rousers and militants, often corrupt or radical in their politics, are responsible for organizing of employees. Lloyd Reynolds gives us some idea why people join unions by stating

> The decision to join is by no means strictly a natural decision. It is probably more like a religious conversion than like deciding to buy a pair of shoes. The worker does not estimate whether the results he will get from the union will be worth the dues he pays. He is confronted with an emotional appeal and urged to take part in a social and political crusade and he finally decides to accept. Moreover, the decision to join is usually not an individualistic decision. The first few workers (in a hospital) who join the union have to make up their own minds. After a nucleus has been secured, however, the growth of the union develops into a mass movement. Most of the workers join because others have done so and hold-outs are gradually brought into line by the pressure of social ostracism (in the hospital).[1]

We often look at unions as a movement. The fact is that most union members do not view the union as a movement, but rather as a means to an end—as a limited purpose, economic institution. What they are looking for is what they cannot presently find in the institution. It is a matter of unfulfilled needs.

Let us review some of the material presented in Chapter One. We found that there is a marked relationship between worker morale and how much employees feel their boss is interested in discussing work problems with the work group. *Their boss is you.* We found that when the supervisor treats subordinates as human beings, there is greater group loyalty and pride. Employees with group loyalty and pride do not need unions to fill their needs. We also learned that by seeing problems through the eyes of the workers, the supervisor can translate employee needs to top management and thereby help arrive at policy decisions that are realistic and satisfy both administration and employees. Policies arrived at in this way will not drive employees into the arms of union organizers. It was also noted that the basic employee desires are for "full appreciation of work done," "feeling in on things," and "sympathetic help on personal problems." When an employee does not feel appreciated, is not in on things (does not know what is going on and most important, does not know about the things that affect his daily work life), or cannot look to his supervisor for empathy, *then that employee will look elsewhere.* The union stands ready to listen, to promise, to take up the battle for unfulfilled employee needs.

We also reviewed the major dissatisfiers in the work area: company policy, administration, supervision, salary, interpersonal relations, and working conditions. These were compared to the major satisfiers: what the employee does, recognition, responsibility, advancement, and achievement. By improving managerial practices and by proper utilization of both people and technology, the supervisor can increase the satisfaction and productivity of employees. *Satisfied and fulfilled employees are not receptive to union organizers.*

THE UNION ORGANIZER

The typical union organizer nas a natural affinity for people, is a good listener, and knows how and at what level to communicate. Chaney and Beech[2] point out some interesting facts about union organizers and sketch this profile:

1. He or she has a natural capacity to like people. A union organizer is a warm, gentle, outgoing person who communicates well and relates effectively to all types of people.
2. He or she has the ability to adapt to the immediate surroundings and warm up to people very quickly.
3. He or she is patient with people. The union organizer realizes that nonunion employees are not immediately sold on organization. Therefore, the organizer makes an ongoing effort to sign up or convince all employees of the values of unionism and collective action.
4. Many labor relations experts have depicted organizers as a combination missionary, salesperson, psychologist.

Elliot Godoff, who was an especially effective organizer and trainer of organizers once told me that he had developed a staff that knows how to approach people. His people no longer talk simply about wages and benefits; they establish a rapport with the workers on a much higher level. They know when to raise the key issue of employee rights. They show workers how to establish their rights, how to meet with management as equals, how to protect themselves as individuals, and how to win identity within the hospital as important human beings. He added that the organizer who merely tells the worker, "You earn twenty cents less than workers at X hospital and, therefore, you should organize," is out of the picture. Management is more sophisticated; they know more about the union than they did before; their approach is different. He thought that his organizers have kept up with this change.

Let me quote from an interview that I was fortunate to have with Mr. Godoff.

> I think that you will probably get reports from the management in the areas where we work that we don't operate the way we did years ago. You are not going to see circulars floating around and a lot of excitement in the very early stages. Some of our best organizers really work for a period of weeks or months to build an organizing committee, and that means that not a single person has yet signed the card or has made any commitment in terms of paper or materials— simply developing a *very close relationship with people* on the following ratio. If it is a hospital, let's say with a thousand workers, then we will aim for a minimum of a sixty-man or woman organizing committee with whom we are going to meet periodically, raise issues, raise questions, get all the vital information about the hospital— the number of people in the units, the division of the departments, how many in each department, the ethnic division, the character of the supervision, who is the son of a bitch among the supervisors that we can hit the hardest— and then to orient them on a question of rights, rights, rights and rights. We say management can give you wage increases, management can give you benefits, management can do a lot of things, but one thing they are not going to give you is rights. When that becomes something that workers feel— it may be very abstract, it may be very vague— but when they feel rights, they will tell you: I haven't got rights; I want rights. And each one imagines it in his own way, but that becomes the greatest strength that the union can muster in any situation.[3]

Now let us look at what one union sets down as a guide for union organizers.[4] Nicholas Zonarich, organizational director of the Industrial Union Department, AFL-CIO, states:

> The organizer has two immediate objectives when he makes his first contacts with the workers at the plant. He is looking for leadership for his campaign and information about the specific problems and complaints of the employees.

There is no blueprint for meeting individual workers and gaining their confidence—conversations can be started in restaurants and bars, through "leads" passed on by other union members, and by acquaintances made through social affairs. If there is any rule at all, it is that contacts are *not* made by suddenly appearing at a plant gate with a leaflet urging employees to sign a union authorization card and mail it to a post office box.

Most organizers are interested primarily in meeting the type of employee who is respected by his fellow-workers and who has influence inside the plant. Getting to know a few of these employees is more important—at this stage—than meeting the maximum number of workers.

Once a potential plant leader has been contacted, it is important to win his confidence and trust. Time spent in developing this leader, answering his questions about the union, and explaining the benefits of collective bargaining will be well worthwhile after the organizing campaign gets underway and this leader becomes a union spokesman inside the plant.

Articulate and respected leaders inside the plant are vital to any campaign, but the representative must use his own judgment in selecting the right people. He must be sure that they are not known as chronic "gripers" or "soreheads" and that they are not motivated simply by a desire for revenge or a driving personal ambition.

In the "perfect" campaign, the organizer will find a leader for every group in the plant—a woman for the female workers, leaders within minority, racial, and national groupings, and spokesmen for the various departments and shifts. Since the "perfect" situation rarely exists, the staff man must develop a leadership group as representative as possible.

Both Godoff and Zonarich make some interesting points to which I direct your attention. Godoff said they look at "the character of the supervision, who is the son of a bitch among the supervisors that we can hit the hardest." Zonarich points out that the organizer must be sure that the leaders are not known as chronic "gripers" or "soreheads" and that they are not motivated simply by a desire for revenge or driving personal ambition. The union is looking for bona fide constituents to use in the organizing drive. Yes, they will latch on to the petty gripes and perceived injustices, but they are also looking closely for supervisors who are an easy mark—those who are not employee-centered, who have not built up group loyalty.

YOUR EMPLOYEES ARE RATING YOU

There is no question that the first-line supervisor is the person most dramatically affected by the organization of employees. The institution itself may be exposed over the years to restrictions on management rights, increased wages, and increased fringe benefits, but in the final analysis the real impact of unionization is felt at the day-to-day level of supervisor-employee intercourse.

The first-line supervisor must understand the key role he or she plays during the organizational drive. The union is keenly interested in and often extremely aware of the day-to-day supervisor-employee relationship, especially the issues of fairness and consistency. If the employees believe that they are not being treated fairly by their supervisor, they will be more interested in the union's carefully presented approach in the area of employee rights. If the supervisor has played favorites—has handled similar cases in different ways for different employees—then that supervisor and that institution are more vulnerable to the organizers' demand for collective power to enforce such consistency and fairness. Employees look carefully at their supervisor's behavior in similar situations, looking for consistency in more cases than looking for the actual punishment. As we have learned earlier, a sympathetic "no" may be more effective than a harsh "yes." Similarly, a sympathetic "no" in one situation will be compared to the "yes" of the prior situation for the test of consistency. If your decision has been different in what may appear to be similar cases, it is important that you make the difference acceptable by sharing the underlying facts of both situations. But beware: if the underlying facts are similar and you still have reached a different decision, you must explain your reasons.

When groups of employees are faced with the choice of voting for or against the union, they often think in terms of their relationship to their supervisors. Critical to that relationship is a supervisor's integrity. How you are perceived by your employees when they are in the voting booth is often a reflection of your actions over the years. Have you truly represented the workers to the management and the management to the workers?

Several suggestions that can produce group loyalty and high productivity (and most important, reflect favorably on your integrity) should be reviewed at this time:

1. Keep employees informed about developments.
2. Recommend pay increases where they are indicated.
3. Keep your people posted on how well they are doing.
4. Take the time to listen, empathetically, to employee complaints and grievances.
5. Permit employees to discuss work problems with you.
6. Recommend employees for promotional opportunities.
7. Don't take all the credit; share the product of your department's labor with all participating and productive members of the team.
8. Display consistent and dependable behavior
9. Discipline in private.
10. Help employees improve and broaden.
11. Treat all members of your department as equals.

Labor unions capitalize on management mistakes. The need for unionization is created by the management rather than the union. If the management (and that includes the first-line supervisor) does not understand or care about employee needs, the union wins the election. It is evident that institutions and supervisors have become increasingly sophisticated and aware of what drives employees into unions

HOW UNIONS HAVE FARED IN ELECTIONS

During the first ten months of the health care industry's inclusion under the National Labor Relations Act (July 1974-April 1975), health care unions won 59.7 percent of the elections as compared with a win record in industry of 47.4 percent. It was clear that the health care industry was more vulnerable to unionization than were other industries at that time. But in the next twelve months (May 1975-April 1976), health care unions won only 58 percent of the elections as compared with a win record in industry of 47.2 percent— a movement, although not dramatic, toward fewer union wins.

In the period from April 1976 through January 1977, 281 elections were conducted in the health services industry. The unions won 132 of these, a win record of only 47 percent. This latest statistic shows the reversal of a trend in which unions were more victorious in the health services industry than in other industries. I believe that we have stopped playing the part of Brutus who looked to the stars for the cause of his misfortune. Rather we have adopted the view of Pogo, "We have met the enemy and they are us." We have looked into ourselves for the root causes of employee unrest and collective action. We have been more pragmatic about our approaches to employee relations, and it is showing.

WHAT YOU CAN AND CANNOT DO DURING A UNION ORGANIZING DRIVE

A committee of the American Bar Association and a committee of publishers and associations included in a declaration of principles that writers who deal with any subject that has or may have legal overtones shall declare that they are not engaged in rendering legal service. *If legal service or other expert assistance is required, the services of a competent professional should be sought.* There is no question that when a union approaches an institution that institution should have sound labor relations and, if necessary, legal advice. But in the final analysis a simple dose of common sense would suffice.

You, the first-line supervisor, will be on the firing line in such a situation. You will have to know what is and is not permissible as far as the National Labor Relations Act is concerned. But given the pressures of the moment and the supervisor-employee relationships that have developed over the years in your department, it may seem strange to deal with legalities at such a time.

Let's refer then to the overall commonsense approach that has been complicated by legal interpretations. There are three basic proscriptions when dealing with employees during a union organizing campaign:

1. Don't threaten them. (I suggest that you not threaten them at other times as well and, therefore, this warning may seem a little redundant in a book on positive employee relations.)
2. Don't promise them any reward for staying out of the union.
3. Don't interrogate them, especially about their preferences. Never ask, "Are you for the union or are you against the union?"

When and if the union approaches employees in your institution, there will be a great deal of pressure put upon supervisors to deliver a vote for management. Ideally, there will be a complete and open discussion of the pros and cons of unionization led by the top management of your institution, directed toward supervisors at every level. You will be tempted to put pressure on the employees to vote against the union. The National Labor Relations Board (NLRB) has set up general guidelines for managerial behavior during a union organizing drive. You may not threaten employees with the loss of their jobs or reduction in their wages; you may not use threatening or intimidating language. Of course, even common sense directs you not to threaten employees in the exercise of their right to support a union.

Although you cannot personally urge an employee to convince other workers to oppose the union, you may tell employees that when a union enters an institution, problems must be directed toward the shop steward, eliminating the one-to-one discussion between employee and the supervisor. You can share with employees the disadvantages of belonging to a union: paying dues and initiation fees, the possibility of loss of income due to strikes, the necessity for picket line duty. Without using threatening language, you may tell employees that the administration does not want a union and that the institution does not need a union.

You cannot promise increased wages, promotions, or benefits if employees reject the union. You can tell the employee that a union will out-promise an employer, but in the final analysis, the union cannot guarantee anything. It must bargain with the employer, and in order to attain benefit levels, must reach agreement with the employer. You may remind the employees of their present benefits and compare these benefits with those in unionized institutions.

Supervisors may not ask employees their personal opinions about the union or what they believe are the feelings of other employees. You cannot call employees away from their work areas into your office to urge them to vote against the union. You cannot systematically visit the homes of employees to urge them to vote against the union.

You, as a supervisor, can tell employees that they do not have to sign union authorization cards and, indeed, do not have to speak to union organizers at their homes if they do not so desire. You can speak to employees individually or in groups at the employees' work station, in the employee cafeteria, or in other areas where employees are accustomed to being. Remember, it is illegal to ask employees what they think about a union, or how they intend to vote, or if they have signed cards or attended union meetings. But it is permissible for you to tell employees why a union is not necessary in your institution. You may continue to operate normally and continue to discipline and discharge as the situation requires, but not for the sole reason that the employee is involved in union activities— although employees are expected to work at their assignments during working hours.

SOLICITATION AND DISTRIBUTION

Many supervisors find themselves perplexed and anxious to take immediate action when employees in their departments come to work wearing buttons that urge employees to vote for a specific union. The following two cases involve hospitals and the issue of union button wearing.

In the first case, St. Joseph Hospital,[5] the National Labor Relations Board *reversed* an administrative law judge's decision in favor of the hospital and its longstanding dress code against employees who wore union buttons. The buttons said, "Vote for Health Care Division, LIUNA, AFL-CIO." The judge had earlier ruled that the action of the hospital was legal in shielding its patients from controversial issues, but the National Labor Relations Board, who reviewed the administrative law judge's decision upon appeal by the union, said under the dress code employees were permitted to wear other buttons such as those designed to observe hospital week and doctor's day as well as a St. Patrick's Day button saying, "Kiss me, I'm Irish." Thus, the Board concluded, the dress code as applied by the hospital merely prohibited the wearing of union insignia and was not designed to protect the patients. Rather the rule was intended to thwart the union-organizing campaign. The hospital was therefore ordered to cease the discriminatory enforcement of its dress code.

In the second case, Baptist Memorial Hospital,[6] the NLRB *sustained* an administrative law judge's decision that the hospital had violated the act by prohibiting its employees from wearing union buttons. The decision observed that such prohibition served no legitimate hospital purpose, because the wearing of United Fund pins was permitted. Therefore, the judge concluded, "The prohibition against wearing union buttons was designed to thwart the union-organizing campaign of the State, County and Municipal Employees Union." The NLRB concurred with the judge's decision and said that discriminatory application of the hospital rule against wearing insignias *other than professional and hospital pins* was a violation of the act and unlawful.

These two decisions point out that the National Labor Relations Board will rule *against* a hospital's rule that permits the wearing of any buttons or insignia other than professional hospital insignia while at the same time prohibits the wearing of union buttons or insignia. If your hospital wishes to legally prohibit employees from wearing union buttons or insignia, it must strictly enforce a rule that authorizes the wearing of professional and hospital pins and insignias only.

What we should understand from the Board's decisions in this area is that the key question is whether the employer's rule is for purposes of efficiency or safety and is nondiscriminatory in nature—that is, is not directed solely against the union's organizing campaign.

The issue of solicitation is most complex. Solicitation includes the attempt by union organizers (employees or nonemployees) to sign up employees and distribute union campaign material. In general, an employer cannot prevent union organizational activities outside working hours even though the activities take place on the employer's property. This rule was first pronounced by the NLRB and approved by the Supreme Court:

> . . . Time outside working hours, whether before or after work, or during luncheon or rest periods, is an employee's time to use as he wishes without unreasonable restraint, although the employee is on company property. It is therefore not within the province of an employer to promulgate and enforce a rule prohibiting union solicitation by an employee outside of working hours, although on company property. Such a rule must be presumed to be an unreasonable impediment to self-organization and, therefore, discriminatory in the absence of evidence that special circumstances make the rule necessary in order to maintain production or discipline.[7]

It has also been held that lunch hours and rest periods are not "working time" despite the fact they may be short or irregularly scheduled and even though employees may be paid for the periods. Past decisions have indicated that an employer can impose a no solicitation rule during working hours so long as the rule is reasonable, necessary for productive operations and not discriminatory. If the rule is valid on its face but is applied in a discriminatory way, or is used as a lever to prevent the workers from exercising their lawful right to organize, the NLRB will call for its elimination.[8]

Another key question is should hospital cafeterias and vending machine areas be off limits to union solicitation or the distribution of union campaign material? The American Hospital Association (AHA) asked the court to justify additional restrictions on employee solicitation and distribution in order to maintain the tranquil atmosphere essential to a hospital's primary function of providing high quality patient care. The opinion appeared in a brief to a most interesting case, St. John's Hospital and School of Nursing.[9]

> . . . All areas of the hospital to which patients have access must be areas which the hospital is entitled to regulate. Additionally we submit the special circumstances which the duties owed to patients and visitors place upon the employer and the employee . . . extend beyond "strictly patient care areas." *They extend throughout the hospital to areas where patients and visitors have access.*

The American Hospital Association maintains that the patient—removed from familiar surroundings and anticipating pain, discomfort, the unknown, and the use of procedures and practices he or she simply does not understand—needs to have considerable and thoughtful support from all personnel involved in the delivery of health care. The AHA asserts that any disruption in that setting (which would include union organizing activities) creates patient anxiety, unrest, or emotional stress.[10] The court ruled that the hospital had the right to prohibit solicitation in its cafeteria and gift shop, both of which are open to the public. The court concluded that the hospital maintains the same commercial interest in its cafeteria and gift shop as is held by the management of retail stores and restaurants located in other types of establishments. The hospital does not lose its right to prohibit solicitation in those facilities, "simply because its public cafeteria and gift shop is a part of the hospital complex rather than a shopping mall or a drive-in restaurant." Of course, *this case pertained only to St. John's.* In a recent Supreme Court ruling [Beth Israel Hospital v. NLRB, No. 77-152 (June 22, 1978)], the Justices unanimously upheld a decision of the NLRB that the Boston hospital could not bar solicitation and distribution of literature in its cafeteria and coffee shop. Although the NLRB has barred such activity in public restaurants, the Court noted that 77 percent of the cafeteria's customers at the hospital were employees, making it "a natural gathering place for distribution of union material." It should be noted that four of the nine Justices agreed with the result, but challenged the general application to hospitals of a 1945 industrial ruling that employer interference with distribution of union literature is presumed to be illegal absent special circumstances. This should give you some idea of the complex nature of the solicitation question. Since this area is highly technical, hospital administration would do well to retain labor counsel.

PERMISSIBLE AND IMPERMISSIBLE CAMPAIGNING

We will once again review what is and is not permissible regarding management action during a union organizing campaign. Various decisions of the National Labor Relations Board in this area have established legal distinctions that govern the rights of management to speak freely when combating a union organizing drive. The following checklist is not all inclusive but is presented to encourage your institution to take a stand during such a period. It cannot be said too often that taking a neutral position or taking no position at all during a union organizing campaign is tantamount to agreeing to the organization of your employees. If the hospital is against recognizing a union, it can and should:

1. Explain the meaning of union recognition and the procedure to be followed.

2. Encourage each member of the bargaining unit (those employees who will be permitted to vote in a union election) to actually cast their ballot in the election.

3. Communicate to employees that they are free to vote for or against the union, despite the fact that they have signed a union authorization card.

4. Communicate to all employees why the administration is against recognizing a union.

5. Review the compensation and benefits program, pointing out the record of the administration in the past.

6. Point out to employees statements made by the union which the administration believes to be untrue, and communicate its own position on each of these statements.

7. If there is a general no solicitation rule, prevent solicitation of membership by the union during working hours.

8. Continue to enforce all rules and regulations in effect prior to the union's request for recognition.

9. Send letters to employees' homes stating the administration's position and record and the administration's knowledge of the union's position in other hospitals.

10. Discuss the possibility of strikes when unions enter hospitals; discuss the ramifications of such a strike.

11. Discuss the impact of union dues and in general the cost of belonging to a union. Point out to the employees that the union can promise the employees anything, but it can deliver on promises only with the agreement of the administration.

12. Discuss with employees, individually at their work areas, the position of the institution.

13. In response to the union's promises during the preelection period, point out to employees that if the hospital were to meet these demands it might be forced to lay off workers. (This statement can be made as long as the administration points out that it would be an involuntary action and a consequence of a union's demands.)

Of course the hospital *cannot* and *should not* engage in the following activities during the union organizing drive:

1. Promise benefits and threaten reprisals if employees vote for or against the union, or have supervisors attend union meetings or spy on employees to determine whether or not they are participating in union activities.
2. Grant wage increases or special concessions during the preelection period unless the timing coincides with well-established prior practices.
3. Prevent employees from wearing union buttons, except in cases where the buttons are provocative or extremely large.
4. Bar employee union representatives from soliciting employee membership during *nonworking hours* when the solicitation does not interfere with the work of others.
5. Summon an employee into an office for private discussion of the union and the upcoming elections. (This does not preclude an employee from coming in voluntarily to discuss these things.)
6. Question employees about union matters and meetings.
7. Ask employees how they intend to vote.
8. Threaten layoffs because of unionization or state that you will never deal with a union even if it is certified.
9. Hold meetings with employees within the 24-hour period immediately preceding the election.[11]

There is much that the employer can say and do during the union organizing campaign. In a health care facility as discussed above, no solicitation and no distribution rules can be enforced if properly constructed and properly administered without discrimination per se against the union and in the interest of maintaining patient care. As we shall see, it is essential that as many qualified members of the employee body—those who are included in the bargaining unit—vote at a time of an election. It has been shown that employees who are eligible to vote but do not vote in the union election would probably vote *against* the union; on the other hand, employees who favor unions will come out to vote. So, as a supervisor you should encourage all employees in your department who are eligible to vote to do so.

It is essential to differentiate between communications that are threatening or carry promises of reward and those designed to bring management's position honestly and forthrightly to all eligible employees. As to the question of free speech, the National Labor Relations Board judges each case on its own merits. The essential element is the "total context" which will determine whether the communication was coercive, threatening, or contained promises. Employees should be told that signing a union authorization card is not equivalent to a vote for the union; the voting will be by secret ballot and an employee can make a *final* decision at that time, notwithstanding the fact that he or she has signed a union authorization card. In an election conducted by a National Labor Relations Board, the marking of ballots is decisive, not the presentation of signed authorization cards.

I repeat an important point made earlier, that I do not contend to render legal service in reviewing this critical and complex area of union organization. If legal service or other expert assistance is deemed necessary by your institution, the services of a competent professional should be sought.

THE BARGAINING UNIT

The bargaining unit is defined as employees who will vote in an election to determine whether or not they wish to be represented by a union. Appropriate bargaining units are determined by the National Labor Relations Board. The health care industry, only recently included under the Taft-Hartley Act, had special problems that were addressed in the deliberations of the congressional committees considering the inclusion of the health care industry in 1974. One of the considerations of the committee was stated in the congressional report:

. . . Due consideration should be given by the (National Labor Relations) Board to prevent the proliferation of bargaining units in the health care industry.

Congress recognized the difficult burden that would be thrust upon health care institutions if various employee groups could form into separate bargaining units, thereby forcing the hospital to negotiate contracts with dozens of unions. The issue of an appropriate bargaining unit is a complex one, but in general you may be dealing with units of:

- service and maintenance employees,
- registered nurses,
- guards,
- technical employees,
- business office clericals,
- MDs, and
- other professionals.

One thing is clear—you, as a supervisor, are *excluded* from the provisions of the act. Therefore, the administration need not recognize a bargaining unit of supervisors; the board may not certify a labor organization seeking to represent supervisors.

Once the bargaining unit is determined, the board will ascertain whether there is an appropriate "show of interest." This show of interest is displayed by the union presenting union authorization cards for at least 30 percent of the bargaining unit employees. Remember, however, although this 30 percent figure will enable the union to obtain an election under National Labor Relations Board auspices, the union needs much more support than that to win the election. (We will cover this later in this chapter.)

THE ELECTION PROCESS

Once having determined that there is a "show of interest," the NLRB will set an election date and determine the time and place for the election. Usually the election will be held on hospital premises. The voting place is determined by mutual agreement between the employer and the union, but final determination is made by the board itself. Present at the polling area is an NLRB representative who is directly responsible for conducting the election. In addition, the union provides an *observer* and the hospital provides an *observer*. The hospital's observer may not be a supervisor.

Within seven days after the NLRB regional director has approved an election, the board is provided with a list of all eligible employees. This list contains the names and addresses of all unit employees. Generally, employees are eligible to vote if they are on the employer's payroll for the period immediately prior to the date on which the election is held. In addition, employees who are engaged in an economic strike and have been permanently replaced are still eligible to vote if the election is held within twelve months of the strike. Employees who are on layoff status but have a "reasonable expectation of reemployment" in the near future have been deemed eligible to vote. Those who have been discharged for cause or who have quit between the date the election was set and the actual voting day are ineligible unless such employees have been discriminatorily discharged.[12]

Employees have the opportunity to vote in secret. They mark a simple ballot *yes* or *no* on the question of whether they wish to be represented by the specific union petitioning. *A union must receive a majority of the valid ballots cast in order to be certified.* If 50 percent plus one employee of the employees who voted in the election cast their ballots in favor of the union, the union will become the certified representative of the bargaining unit for the purposes of collective bargaining.

A simple illustration will underscore the importance of getting out the vote. If a bargaining unit of 500 service and maintenance employees at your institution is involved in an election, the union must receive a majority of the valid ballots cast. If only 400 of these employees actually vote, the union need only receive 201 votes. As you can plainly see, if 201 out of 400 voting employees cast their ballots for the union, the union will be certified to represent all 500 employees in the bargaining unit. The 100 employees who did not vote have no effect on the outcome of the election. Remember, many presidents of the United States have been elected by a majority of the votes cast, but by a significant *minority* of the eligible electorate. *So go union elections.*

Key Points in a Union Organizing Drive

1. More employees vote for or against their immediate supervisor than for or against top management, the board of trustees, or consultants.

2. Unions rarely organize employees; rather, it is administration's poor record in employee relations that drives employees into unions.

3. Institutions that provide all the benefits and conditions of the union shop will not become unionized.

4. There is a marked relationship between worker morale and the extent to which employees feel their boss is interested in discussing work problems with their work group. If the boss—*that's you!*—is not interested, workers will discuss those problems with outside groups—*in some cases, unions.*

5. Employees who feel group loyalty and pride do not look outside to unions for need fulfillment.

6. Improved managerial practices and the supervisor's attention to the best utilization of people and technology can increase job satisfaction and productivity. *Satisfied and fulfilled employees do not look to unions.*

7. Unions are looking for bona fide issues to use in the organizing drive. Although they will latch on to petty gripes and perceived injustices, they often look for supervisors who are vulnerable. Such supervisors are usually not employee-centered, have not built up group loyalty, and are not interested in employee needs.

8. Labor unions capitalize on management mistakes.

9. You should not threaten employees or promise them any reward for staying out of the union. Do not interrogate them about their preferences during a union organizing drive. These are unfair labor practices.

10. You can tell employees how the institution feels about unionization. You can share with them the employee disadvantages of belonging to a union.

11. You cannot call employees away from their work areas into your office in order to urge them to vote against the union.

12. You should tell employees that they do not have to sign union authorization cards or speak to union organizers if they do not so desire.

13. You should inform employees that even though they have signed a union authorization card, *they can change their mind* and vote any way they wish at the time of an election.

14. You should encourage each member of your department who is in the bargaining unit (those employees eligible to vote) to actually cast a ballot in the election.

15. You should continue to enforce all rules and regulations in effect prior to the union's request for recognition.

16. You should keep top management apprised of day-to-day developments during the union organizing campaign. You will be the person closest to the employees at that time. Your perception of trends is critical to administration planning.

17. Recent statistics indicate that unions win only 47 percent of elections in the health care industry. This is a reversal of earlier statistics obtained during the first year of the industry's coverage under the Taft-Hartley Act. The reversal indicates a more sophisticated and concerned management approach toward employee needs.

NOTES

1. Lloyd Reynolds, *Labor Economics and Labor Relations* (Englewood Cliffs, N.J.: Prentice-Hall, Inc., 1956), p. 60.

2. Warren H. Chaney and Thomas R. Beech, *The Union Epidemic* (Germantown, Md.: Aspen Systems Corporation, 1976), pp. 45-46.

3. From an interview with Elliot Godoff conducted by Norman Metzger on February 29, 1972. The late Mr. Godoff was Executive Vice President/Organization Director of District 1199, Drug and Hospital Union.

4. *A Guidebook for Union Organizers,* Industrial Union Department, AFL-CIO, Distributed by Master Printers of America, Washington, D.C.

5. St. Joseph Hospital, 225 NLRB 28, 16 CA 6019, Fort Worth, Tex., June 30, 1976

6. Baptist Memorial Hospital, 225 NLRB 69, 26 CA 5743, 5781, 5875, Memphis, Tenn., June 30, 1976.

7. Republic Aviation v. NLRB, 324 US 793, 65 S. Ct. 982.

8. *Ground Rules for Labor and Management during Organizing Drives* (Englewood Cliffs. N.J.: Prentice-Hall, Inc., 1970), p. 22.

9. St. John's Hospital and School of Nursing, Inc. v. NLRB, CA 10, 82 LC, paragraph 10,021.

10. Brief of the American Hospital Association, Amicus Curiae, St. John's Hospital and School of Nursing, Inc. v. NLRB, *Ibid.*

11. Norman Metzger and Dennis Pointer, *Labor Management Relations in the Health Service Industry: Theory and Practice* (Washington, D.C.: Science and Health Publications, Inc., 1972), pp. 143-144.

12. Dennis Pointer and Norman Metzger, *The National Labor Relations Act: A Guidebook for Health Care Facility Administrators* (New York: Spectrum Publications, Inc., 1975), pp. 72-73.

Chapter 9

How to Measure Results of Your Supervisory Efforts

Peter Drucker, a leading management thinker on the role of the modern manager, states in the beginning of one of his books,

> To be effective is the job of the executive. "To effect" and "to execute" are, after all, near-synonyms. Whether he works in a business or in a hospital, in a government agency or in a labor union, in a university or in the army, the executive is, first of all, expected to get the *right things done.* And this is simply that he is expected to be effective.[1]

Although Drucker uses the term "simply that he is expected to be effective," it is not a *simple* matter to measure effectiveness. You, as a supervisor, must first know what is expected of you; you depend on another strata of management (the department head) to communicate clearly the goals of the organization and the objectives for your department.

Management by objective programs would be of inordinate help in evaluating your effectiveness and more importantly, coming to agreement on that evaluation. The advance communication of clear, important, and relevant goals and the establishment of priorities for those goals have been shown to improve the subordinate's efficiency and the relationship between subordinates and superiors. In a study of the subject, Caroll and Tosi found that subordinates are positive toward the program (management by objectives) when it helps them to clarify and gain agreement on what is expected of them.[2]

SETTING OF GOALS

The real key is the setting of the goals. Evaluating performance against those goals is facilitated by a clear definition of the goal and the way in which the goal is established and communicated. It is of critical importance that you concentrate on the quality of the goals and the goal-setting mechanism, that you convince your superiors of the importance of your participation in that procedure.

Kay offers the following guidelines for setting better quality goals:

1. A goal implies some achievement as a result of a subordinate's doing something. The initial step in clarifying a goal is to begin with "to" followed by a verb: to reduce, to provide, to identify.

2. Each goal should relate to a single *end result.* This pinpoints what is expected and also permits more specific measurement— for example, "to reduce turnover by 10 percent by the end of the fourth quarter." The end result in this case is the reduction of turnover. This goal can be further clarified by specifying the area(s) where turnover will be reduced: "to reduce turnover in area B-7 by 10 percent by the end of the fourth quarter."

3. The measurement should be stated in quantitative terms insofar as possible. For turnover reduction the quantitative measurement is a 10 percent reduction. This, of course, implies the availability of turnover data for an agreed upon base period against which the measurement will be taken. Some goals are difficult to specify quantitatively— for example, "to improve the quality of field service manuals." The key question is, "What is a better quality manual?" Is it more readable, shorter, longer, with more or fewer illustrations? What is meant by "better quality" is something that the superior and the subordinate should discuss and specify in as much detail as possible *in advance* of the work being done. In such situations a superior might provide sample material as an example of "better quality" features.

4. The goal should specify when the end result will be achieved. In the example above the end result will be met by the end of the fourth quarter. This helps the subordinate structure time before the due date. It enables the superior and subordinate to measure progress in reaching the end result and signals a review of the total spot.[3]

If you are expected to work toward the attainment of institutional goals, then the institution must incorporate your input into the establishment of such goals. The measurement and appraisal of supervisory performances has been mired in the structure of appraisal systems. Too often reliance on so-called rating systems for supervisory effectiveness has produced a stereotyped report not plugged into overall institutional goals. Such nebulous traits as "cooperation with management," "personal relationships," and "initiative," often result in ratings that produce arguments and differences of opinion rather than constructive evaluations. Mechanical policing methods are not the answer. You want to know exactly what the institution and specifically what the department head expects from you; how your effectiveness is going to be measured; what the department head thinks of you; how well you have measured up to the department head's expectations; and finally, how well you did as measured against the agreed upon goals and objectives of your department.

In Chapter Four we discussed your responsibility for evaluating the performance of employees in your department. Much of that discussion pertains to the evaluation of your own effectiveness. The management by objective process was described briefly in that chapter. The following short review will focus attention on the evaluation of your own effectiveness.

Management by objectives was defined by George S. Odiorne as "a process whereby the superior and the subordinate managers of an enterprise jointly identify the common goals, define each individual's major area of responsibility in terms of the results expected of him, and use these measures as guides for operating the unit and assessing the contribution of members."[4]

As you can see, your commitment to the objectives of the organization depends on your participation in framing those goals so that they are indeed common ones against which your performance can be measured quantitatively and qualitatively. Ideally, you and your superior will perceive the goals of the organization and your own individual goals as essentially the same, taking into account differences in shade or emphasis. Given such agreement, you can derive satisfaction from moving toward the goals of the organization. The key then is to integrate the goals of the institution, subordinates, and management.

MANAGEMENT EFFECTIVENESS

Likert identified three variables useful in discussing management effectiveness: causal, intervening, and end result.[5] Causal variables are leadership strategies, skills and behavior, management's decisions, and the policies and structure of the organization. Intervening variables are the commitment to objectives, motivation and morale of members, their skills and leadership communications, conflict resolution, decision making, and problem solving. Output or end result variables are the dependent variables that reflect the achievements of the organization. *Likert stated that more than 90 percent of managers in organizations look at output alone,* but it is essential that we carefully separate long-term from short-term goals. A narrow concentration on short-term goals may thwart the long-term objectives of building good relationships and developing a stable and productive work force. Most of us are prone to emphasize output variables such as departmental production, budgets, union-management relations, and turnover. But leadership effectiveness takes into account communication, conflict resolution, decision making, and problem solving, along with boosting the motivation and morale of the employees in your department. It is essential that you not judge your effectiveness in too limited a vein.

Too many managers believe the effectiveness of a supervisor's performance can be easily measured. They refer to such measurements as manhours, budgeted versus actual; units of production; absenteeism and lateness; turnover. These benchmarks should neither be underestimated nor overestimated. But we must look beyond these obvious factors to the *immeasurables.* It is a mistake to direct our attention only to areas of supervisory performance that can be measured in statistical terms, or quantified. The key question must be "Is the supervisor building an organization *today* that will meet the needs of the institution *tomorrow?*" Such factors as employee morale, loyalty to the group and to the institution, acceptance of the goals of the institution, pride in the work being done and in the institution itself, trust in the supervisor— all these things are often impossible to measure. The day-to-day pressures inherent in a health care institution too often accentuate the measurable and underestimate the immeasurable factors of supervisory effectiveness.

This situation is further aggravated by the phenomenon of *bottom-line* management. With the complicated and critical issue of third party reimbursement looming heavily over most health care facilities, managers are hard-pressed to meet budgets at any cost— make the bottom line. Pressures develop over choosing which expense will be reduced and which service will be compromised. These needs are real and important, but in focusing attention on the bottom line, supervisors may lose sight of the fact that *organizations are people.* An effective supervisor is one who can meet bottom-line expectations and at the same time maintain high employee morale. Although authoritarian leadership has produced effective results in meeting bottom-line requirements, it is only through a participatory, democratic approach to leadership that a concomitant responsibility of the supervisor can be fulfilled: maintaining high employee morale.

Your job as a supervisor is to develop what has been called a climate of orderly freedom. Your subordinates must feel free to speak up, to make suggestions, to explain differences, to participate in decision making. This of course does not mean that you should abdicate your role as a leader. As a leader you are the individual who can effectively guide group activities toward goal setting and goal achievement.

A CAREER IN MANAGEMENT

To understand the guideposts that mark a successful career in management, we should look to what managers consider important indicators of career satisfaction: what they think has added to progress in their careers, what has detracted from that progress, and finally, what factors produce pressure and stress.

A study conducted by Pearse for the American Management Association looked into these questions.[6] Managers in the middle strata of the management team list as significant to their satisfaction such factors as: recognition for their efforts, contributions, accomplishments, a job well done; the opportunity to demonstrate personal competence; the opportunity to do work that is personally meaningful; and the opportunity to tackle difficult problems in challenging situations. It is clear that *recognition for a job well done* is as significant to managers as it is to subordinates. Managers best guage their success and effectiveness by noting how their supervisors at the next level perceive them. Doing the job well is just not enough. Someone at the top must recognize the success of the effort.

Middle managers see the following factors as most likely to result in steady advancement: proved ability to lead and motivate others; achievement of high-level individual results; proved ability to come up with creative and innovative ideas and methods. Although the last two factors were mentioned by many, the first factor was the only one which a majority of middle management identified. It is clear that most modern managers believe that leadership and the ability to motivate others are critical to a successful managerial career.

Finally, Pearse's study identified factors most likely to impede future career advancement. Middle managers listed the following factors: fewer managerial jobs resulting from organizational streamlining; being too closely identified with a particular organizational faction or power group; inadequate career planning and guidance; lack of own adequate managerial talents and/or professional skills. Pearse concluded that middle managers believe that their own individual efforts, abilities, and activities have much to do with overcoming possible advancement blocks, and they are particularly aware that social and organizational

factors have just as strong an influence on future advancement opportunities.[7]

SUPERVISORY PRACTICES ASSOCIATED WITH
SUPERVISORY EFFECTIVENESS

Study after study indicates that certain supervisory practices will
result in high productivity and high job satisfaction, which can be defined
as effective supervision. These practices include:

1. the use of an open approach—understanding of feelings, building
leadership on the basis of motivational skills;
2. the practice of developing close personal interest in subordinates;
3. a display of sensitivity to the needs of subordinates on a "feelings"
level;
4. the development and continued awareness of group processes;
knowing which supervisory practices produced pride in the group and
loyalty to fellow workers and to the group;
5. the use of a supervisory style that permits freedom and latitude;
general supervision rather than close supervision; and
6. the encouragement of participation and sharing in decisions by
subordinates.

Likert's studies[8] indicate that there is a clear difference in supervision
as it is practiced by supervisors of highly productive units and supervisors of unproductive units. In reviewing seven essential supervisory
practices, the studies showed that the real difference in effectiveness was
not in the standard production-oriented tasks, but rather in the people-
oriented practices such as recommending promotions, transfers, pay increases, informing subordinates on what is happening in the institution,
keeping subordinates posted on how well they are doing, and, finally,
hearing complaints and grievances. When work groups with the highest
and lowest morale are asked to describe what their supervisors did, the
workers in low morale groups mention *just as often* as workers in high
morale groups that the supervisors performed such production-oriented
tasks as "enforces the rules," "arranges work and makes work assignments," and "supplies men with materials and tools." But the high
morale groups mention much *more frequently* than the low morale
groups such employee-centered functions as "recommends promotions
and pay increases," "informs men of what is happening in the company,'
"keeps men posted on how well they are doing," and "hears complaints
and grievances."

CONCLUSION

The effectiveness of a supervisor must be measured within the context of *the other pay system.* Preoccupation with the regular pay system has led to the gross dissatisfaction of workers. This discontent manifests itself in low efficiency, uncooperativeness, and antisocial behavior. The effective supervisor works every day to develop an atmosphere that motivates the employee to work toward the accomplishment of institutional goals and at the same time satisfy his or her own needs for recognition, appreciation, fulfillment, and dignity.

Most research studies seem to come up with a universal finding: *workers want to be loyal to their institution.* Poor supervisory practices breed discontent; sound supervisory practices will enhance that desire to be loyal. Cooperation, participation, and clear and constant communication are vital. High morale is achieved when your subordinates feel the institution is interested in them and their ideas. It also results from individual and group participation where there is a clear indication that their supervisor is listening. Supervisors rated effective by subordinates and who, more often than not, are considered best qualified for promotion, *meet, listen, and consider employee needs, suggestions, and general input.*

Your leadership style has the single greatest effect on your group's productivity and growth. Leader dominance— often misunderstood as leader effectiveness— can result in group apathy, while group participation and group thinking will encourage creativity.

The effective supervisor will more often than not do the following:

1. Keep employees informed of work requirements.
2. Let the employee know where he or she stands.
3. Attain maximum participation and use maximum communication when changes are indicated.
4. Help the employee improve and broaden his or her skills.
5. Compliment the employee for a job well done.
6. Provide the opportunity for group and individual participation in solving work problems.
7. Treat all members of the group as equals.
8. Delegate responsibilities and encourage the acceptance of these responsibilities by all members in the department.
9. Understand each employee's job and clarify the importance of each job in relationship to the group.
10. Appreciate and attempt to solve and/or alleviate employees' problems, no matter how minute.

11. Help the individual understand the basic reasoning and management thinking behind the things he or she is required to do.

Significant results cannot be accomplished solely by power, prestige, and authority. The real power a supervisor has is achieved through a network of satisfactory relationships. Genuine authority is born and nurtured out of respect your people feel you are giving them and the understanding you have for their problems. In your role as liaison between workers and top management, in your role as representing your people to top management and top management to your people, you need to become conscious of three factors:

- the goals of the institution,
- the needs and interests of the workers,
- your own needs and goals.

Effective supervision can result only from a *full appreciation of all three factors*. An institution which affords recognition of an employee as he relates to that institution—a full recognition of the employee's functions and importance—such an institution will promote good morale, purposeful motivation, and increased productivity. The person most responsible for building that climate is the first-line supervisor.

This book ends as it began, by pointing out that if you are going to succeed in the modern work area with its complex challenges produced by changes in our society, higher expectations from employees and a more educated work group, then you must move from an authority-obedience style of supervision to one characterized by involvement, participation, and commitment.

NOTES

1. Peter F. Drucker, *The Effective Executive* (New York: Harper and Row, 1966), p. 1.

2. J. C. Caroll and H. L. Tosi, Jr., *Management by Objectives: Applications and Research* (New York: MacMillan, 1973), passim.

3. Emanuel Kay, *The Crisis in Middle Management* (New York: AMA-COM, A Division of American Management Association, 1974), pp. 103-104.

4. George S. Odiorne, *Management by Objectives: A System of Managerial Leadership* (New York: Pittman Publishing Company, 1965), p. 78.

5. Rensis Likert, *New Patterns of Management* (New York: McGraw-Hill Book Company, 1961), pp. 2-12.

6. Robert F. Pearse, *Manager to Manager II: What Managers Think of Their Managerial Careers* (New York: AMA-COM, A Division of American Management Association, 1977), pp. 25-27.

7. Ibid., pp. 25-31.

8. Rensis Likert, *Motivation: The Core of Management* (New York: American Management Association, Personnel Series No. 155, 1953), p. 9.

Supervisors' Checklist: It's Time To Take Inventory*

CHECKLIST A: FOR DEPARTMENT HEAD LEVEL

This soul-searching exercise is directed toward key management personnel in health care facilities who are responsible for entire departments and, therefore, have other levels of supervision reporting to them. It is a review of some of the material covered earlier and some of the questions posed in Chapter One. It is a good idea to ask yourself these questions periodically throughout the year.

1. Do you as a department head set the pace and attitudes for your people?
2. Do your people share the job of developing goals?
3. Do you share with your people the goals of the insitution?
4. Do you give your people a sense of direction, something to strive for and achieve?
5. Does each member of your department understand the relationship and importance of his or her individual job to the department's operations and to the institution's operations?
6. Do the people in your department understand their responsibilities?
7. Do you endorse the management theory that if subordinates are to plan their course intelligently and work efficiently they need to know the where, what, and why of their jobs: where they are going, what they are doing, and why they are doing it?
8. Do your subordinates have a feeling of being "in" on things?
9. Do you share information or do you keep secrets?
10. Are the supervisors who report to you familiar with top management's thinking, the latest institutional-wide developments, and the

---

* The author wishes to acknowledge the work of Dr. Leslie M. Slote, industrial psychologist, Hartsdale, N.Y., who developed many of the suggestions for supervisory practices at the various levels.

relative importance of various departmental activities to the institution's short- and long-range plans?

11. Do you recogize and accept that it is your responsibility and a priority obligation to keep everyone in your department informed of institutional policy, day-to-day decisions, and most important, reasons for change that affects them as individuals and as work groups?

12. Do your supervisors understand and accept the institution's goals and know how to motivate their subordinates to achieve those goals?

13. Do you notify your people ahead of time of impending changes?

14. Do your requests to your subordinates include the reasons for the requests?

15. Do you have an accurate feedback mechanism?

16. Do you know how your people react to your decisions?

17. Do you know how your people perceive you and the administration?

18. Are you able to cope with rapidly changing situations?

19. Are you able to replan, reorganize, and take emergency action when indicated?

20. Do you have confidence in the people who work for you?

21. Do you indicate such confidence by delegating responsibility with appropriate authority?

22. Are your actions consistent?

23. Are your actions predictable?

24. Do you recognize effort and good work?

25. Do you recognize poor effort and attempt to correct it promptly?

26. Are you convinced that it is just as easy to be positive as to be negative?

27. Do you realize that praise and encouragement often are more productive than criticism?

28. Do your employees feel free to bring problems to you?

29. Have you established a receptive atmosphere for hearing and acting on employee complaints and suggestions?

30. Are you developing understudies from your immediate management level?

31. Is there someone in the department who can replace you if you leave?

32. Do you have a carefully considered supervisory selection and training program for obtaining and developing the type of supervision you want?

33. Do you hold a good person down in one position because he or she is so indispensable there?

34. Do you take a chance on your people by letting them learn through mistakes, by showing a calm reaction and constructive approach to occasional failure, by encouraging them to stick their necks out without fear of the ax, and by instilling self-confidence?

35. Do you use every opportunity to build up in subordinates a sense of the importance of their work?

36. Are you giving real responsibility to your immediate supervisors and then holding them accountable?

37. Do you interfere with jobs of subordinates or do you allow them to exercise discretion and judgment in making decisions?

38. Are you doing things to discourage your subordinates?

39. Are you interested in and aware of the sources of discontentment or discouragement or frustration affecting your supervisors?

40. Do you encourage and listen to the ideas and reactions of your subordinates?

41. Do you give your subordinates credit for their contributions?

42. Do you explain to them why their ideas or suggestions are not acceptable?

43. Do you remember to praise in public but criticize in private?

44. Do you do criticize constructively?

45. Are you aware that a feeling of belonging builds self-confidence and makes people want to work harder than ever?

46. Do you show your people a future?

47. Are you aware of the fact that maximum self-development always takes place when a person feels, understands, accepts, and exercises the full weight of responsibility for his or her job?

CHECKLIST B: FOR INTERMEDIATE-LEVEL SUPERVISORS

You are in a position where you report to a department head and have first-line supervisors reporting to you. Refer to this checklist throughout the year to gauge your effectiveness.

1. Do you have a thorough understanding of institutional goals, your part in meeting budgets, and do you have full confidence in their attainment?

2. Do you offer suggestions or constructive criticism to your supervisor (the department head) and ask for additional information when necessary?

3. Do you build team spirit and group pride by getting everyone into the act of setting goals and pulling together?

4. Do you deal with emergencies as they come up or do you have scheduled times for meetings with your department head and with your first-line supervisors?

5. Do you encourage each of your supervisors to come up with suggestions on ways to improve things?

6. When you do not accept your supervisors' suggestions, do you explain why?

7. Have you set up an atmosphere that enables your subordinates to approach you with job or personal problems?

8. Do people believe that you listen empathetically and really care about their problems?

9. Do you keep your supervisors informed on how they are doing?

10. Do you give credit where credit is due and offer constructive criticism when necessary?

11. Do your supervisors appear to be too busy with work problems to be concerned about their employees' personal difficulties?

12. Does your example encourage your supervisors to build individual worker confidence and praise good performance?

13. Do your supervisors know that you expect them to communicate to their people how jobs are evaluated and what the job rates and progressions are?

14. Do your supervisors keep their people informed of promotional opportunities?

15. Do your supervisors train their people for better jobs?

CHECKLIST C: FOR IMMEDIATE/FIRST-LINE SUPERVISORS

As a first-line supervisor you should review the following checklist on a regular basis.

1. Do you know that good communication means being available to answer employee questions?

2. Do you accept employees' need to know what is expected of them, how well they are doing their jobs, and how they will be rewarded for good work?

3. Have you permitted your employees freedom and latitude in performing their work, or are you constantly supervising employees?

4. Are you personally interested in the well-being of the people who work for you?

5. Do you recommend good workers for promotions, merit increases, and other forms of recognition?

6. Do you consult with your employees and permit them to share in the decision-making process?

7. Do you realize that pent-up emotions are dangerous and, therefore, do you provide an accessible sounding board for employee complaints and grievances?

8. Do you ever say or do anything that detracts from the sense of personal dignity that each of your people has?

9. When a job is well done do you praise the worker, and when a job is done poorly do you criticize constructively?

10. Do you realize that people want to feel important?

11. Do you realize that people want recognition?

12. Do you realize that people want credit and attention?

13. Do you realize that people have their own self-interest at heart?

14. Do you realize that people want to be better off tomorrow than today?

15. Do you realize that people want prompt action on their questions?

16. Do you realize that people would rather talk than listen?

17. Do you realize that people would rather give advice than take advice?

18. Do you realize that people generally resent too-close supervision?

19. Do you realize that people resent change?

20. Do you realize that people are naturally curious?

21. Do you ask questions instead of giving orders?

22. Do you make suggestions instead of giving orders?

23. Do you keep in mind the employees' self-interest?

24. Do you make your employees feel that their work is useful?

25. Do you make your employees feel that they are trusted members of the work group?

26. Do you represent your employees' interests to the next level of supervision?

27. Do you represent the management to your employees?

28. Are you too busy with work problems to be concerned with employees' personal difficulties?

29. Do you look for and find opportunities to praise and reward a good performance, or are you afraid of being accused of sentimentality and coddling?

30. Are you consistent or do you play favorites?

31. Are you predictable or do your employees feel they never know what your next move will be?

32. Do you try to rotate your people and build up skills for individual flexibility within the group?

33. Do you spend enough time training your people?

34. Do you understand the problem with legislating change rather than selling change?

35. Do your employees perceive you as a "people-centered" supervisor?

36. Do your employees trust you?

Supervisor Evaluation

Would you dare ask your employees to complete this survey rating you as a supervisor? How would you rate yourself?

1. Supervisor's relationship with his/her staff: Well liked and respected ( ), Usually gets along well with others and makes fair impression ( ), Seldom attracts respect from others ( ), Creates antagonism ( ).

2. Work knowledge of supervisor: Excellent ( ), Good ( ), Fair ( ), I know more than him/her ( ).

3. Does he/she set a good example? Always ( ), Sometimes ( ), If I used him/her as an example I'd be fired ( ).

4. Does he/she provide motivation? Yes ( ) No ( )

5. Do you receive respect? Yes ( ) No ( )

6. Are you dealt with honestly? Yes ( ) No ( )

7. Do you receive praise on a job well done? Yes ( ) No ( )

8. Are you criticized when you perform poorly? Yes ( ) No ( )
Is this criticism beneficial? Yes ( ) No ( )

9. Are you encouraged to take initiative? Yes ( ) No ( )

10. Are you encouraged to make suggestions? Yes ( ) No ( )

11. Is your supervisor too demanding? Yes ( ) No ( )

12. Are schedules and job assignments made fairly? Yes ( ) No ( )

13. Do you feel your supervisor plays favorites? Yes ( ) No ( )

14. Do you feel you were adequately oriented to your job? Yes ( ) No ( )

15. Do you feel your supervisor is willing to help with work if your team is shorthanded? Yes ( ) No ( )

16. Do you feel your supervisor has a heavy work load? Yes ( ) No ( )

17. If you want to speak with your supervisor
will he/she find the time?   Yes ( )   No ( )

18. Do you feel your supervisor will listen with
an open mind?   Yes ( )   No ( )

19. Does your supervisor accept criticism?   Yes ( )   No ( )

20. Do you feel lines of communication are open
above your supervisor?   Yes ( )   No ( )

21. Do unresolved problems with your super-
visor reflect on his/her attitude toward you?   Yes ( )   No ( )

22. Are problems usually worked out?   Yes ( )   No ( )

23. Do you feel your supervisor will stand behind
you when you are right?   Yes ( )   No ( )

24. Do you feel your supervisor cares about your
personal feelings and problems?   Yes ( )   No ( )

List of Authors

Index

About the Author

Norman Metzger is Vice-President for Personnel of the Mount Sinai Medical Center in New York City. In addition, he is a professor of administrative medicine at the Mount Sinai School of Medicine. He is an adjunct associate professor at the Bernard M. Baruch College of the City University of New York in the Department of Management and the graduate program in Health Care Administration. He is, as well, on the faculty of The New School for Social Research and Rensselaer Polytechnic Institute.

Mr. Metzger is a director of the League of Voluntary Hospitals and Homes of New York and was president of the league from 1967 to 1972.

He has written numerous articles on labor relations, personnel administration, and social behavior. He is a two-time recipient of the annual award for literature given by the American Society for Hospital Personnel Administration in recognition of his outstanding contribution to the literature on hospital personnel administration. He is the author of the books:

Personnel Administration in the Health Services Industry: Theory and Practice
The Personnel Function in Health Care Facilities: Personnel Management and Labor Relations (in publication)

and co-author with Dennis Pointer of three books:

Labor-Management Relations in the Health Services Industry: Theory and Practice
The National Labor Relations Act: A Guidebook for Health Care Facility Administrators
Labor Relations and Personnel Management in Long-Term Health Care Facilities